100 Questions & Answers About Your Child's Substance Abuse

Romulo A. Aromin, Jr., MD

Medical Director
Child and Adolescent Partial Hospital Programs
Adolescent MICA
Trinitas Regional Medical Center
Elizabeth, NJ

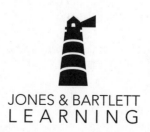

JONES & BARTLETT
LEARNING

World Headquarters

Jones & Bartlett Learning
40 Tall Pine Drive
Sudbury, MA 01776
978-443-5000
info@jblearning.com
www.jblearning.com

Jones & Bartlett Learning
Canada
6339 Ormindale Way
Mississauga, Ontario L5V 1J2
Canada

Jones & Bartlett Learning
International
Barb House, Barb Mews
London W6 7PA
United Kingdom

Jones & Bartlett Learning books and products are available through most bookstores and online booksellers. To contact Jones & Bartlett Learning directly, call 800-832-0034, fax 978-443-8000, or visit our website, www.jblearning.com.

Substantial discounts on bulk quantities of Jones & Bartlett Learning publications are available to corporations, professional associations, and other qualified organizations. For details and specific discount information, contact the special sales department at Jones & Bartlett Learning via the above contact information or send an email to specialsales@jblearning.com.

The author, editor, and publisher have made every effort to provide accurate information. However, they are not responsible for errors, omissions, or for any outcomes related to the use of the contents of this book and take no responsibility for the use of the products and procedures described. Treatments and side effects described in this book may not be applicable to all people; likewise, some people may require a dose or experience a side effect that is not described herein. Drugs and medical devices are discussed that may have limited availability controlled by the Food and Drug Administration (FDA) for use only in a research study or clinical trial. Research, clinical practice, and government regulations often change the accepted standard in this field. When consideration is being given to use of any drug in the clinical setting, the healthcare provider or reader is responsible for determining FDA status of the drug, reading the package insert, and reviewing prescribing information for the most up-to-date recommendations on dose, precautions, and contraindications, and determining the appropriate usage for the product. This is especially important in the case of drugs that are new or seldom used.

Production Credits

Executive Publisher: Christopher Davis
Editorial Assistant: Sara Cameron
Associate Production Editor: Laura Almozara
Associate Marketing Manager: Katie Hennessy
Manufacturing and Inventory Control Supervisor:
  Amy Bacus
Composition: Spoke & Wheel
Printing and Binding: Malloy, Inc.

Cover Credits

Cover Design: Carolyn Downer
Cover Images: Top photo: © Maureen Plainfield/Dreamstime.com; Bottom left photo: © Raisa Kanareva/ShutterStock, Inc.; Bottom right photo: © Andrey Shadrin/ShutterStock, Inc.
Cover Printing: Malloy, Inc.

Library of Congress Cataloging-in-Publication Data

Aromin, Romulo A.
  100 questions and answers about your child's substance abuse / Romulo A. Aromin.
    p. cm.
  title: Hundred questions and answers about your child's substance abuse
  title: One hundred questions and answers about your child's substance abuse
  Includes bibliographical references and index.
  ISBN-13: 978-0-7637-7981-8
  ISBN-10: 0-7637-7981-4
  1. Children—Substance use—Miscellanea. 2. Children—Substance use—Popular works. I. Title. II. Title: Hundred questions and answers about your child's substance abuse. III. Title: One hundred questions and answers about your child's substance abuse.
  RJ506.D78A76 2012
  618.92'.86—dc22

                          2010036987

6048

Printed in the United States of America
14 13 12 11 10   10 9 8 7 6 5 4 3 2 1

To Larry, my family, and my friends.

CONTENTS

Few illnesses bring more fear to a parent than alcoholism and drug abuse. But unlike other disorders that can also be devastating to a child and his or her family, addiction feels particularly confusing— and somehow personal. Where did we go wrong? How did she use all this time without us knowing? Where did he even get the drugs? Okay, I'm ready to accept that what happened happened; so can I help, or am I going to make things even worse?

For other physical and mental illnesses, parents routinely turn to medical specialists for advice and expect guidance and typically follow the experts' recommendations. The very process of charting a course of action with a doctor has significant therapeutic effects for both the child and the parents. Unfortunately, we have come to expect much less from the medical community when it comes to the prevention, diagnosis, and treatment of substance use disorders.

On one hand, we don't trust that we know all that much about the illness itself. Both science and popular culture keep shifting their opinion on the "true" cause of addiction. In the 1960s and the 1970s, it was all about parenting; in the 1980 and the 1990s, we woke up to the monumental discoveries of genetics; and during the past decade, we have been greatly attracted to co-occurring psychiatric disorders including posttraumatic stress disorder, bipolar disorder, attention-deficit hyperactivity disorder, and autism. Recently, family system considerations for both prevention and treatment have resurfaced, bringing us full circle to the world of our parents. Scientists now know that what causes one kid to get drunk and another to stay sober is rather complex. A number of interrelated biological, psychological, and social determinants affect the pleasure, reward, motivation, and memory brain neuronal circuitry leading to impairment in behavioral control, craving, and diminished recognition of significant problems in one's life.

On the other hand, there are very few medical doctors with the appropriate training to address substance use among children and adolescents. The American Board of Psychiatry and Neurology has certified less than 250 psychiatrists in the subspecialty of addiction psychiatry over the past 10 years. Only a handful of these doctors are also board certified in the treatment of children and adolescents. Among this elite group of experts, Dr. Romulo Aromin is one of the very best.

The book that you hold in your hands is Dr. Aromin's straightforward answers to every parent's questions about preventing, identifying, and treating substance abuse and dependence. Based on his extensive scholarship and clinical experience, Dr. Aromin has distilled our current medical knowledge to a small set of practical and easily understood guidelines for parents. While explaining what gateway drugs are, showing us how we can best talk to our children about marijuana, describing in detail anabolic–androgenic steroids and frequently abused prescription pills, warning about the potential pitfalls of home drug testing, and advising on the most effective current treatments, Dr. Aromin avoids medical jargon and maintains an informal yet always scientifically rigorous style. He offers simple and frank suggestions without shying away from the toughest questions. In the end, the answers to the 100 questions addressed in this book form an invaluable manual for sifting through the treacherous, and often murky, waters of substance use in adolescence. The clarity that emerges from Dr. Aromin's work is both highly accessible and greatly appreciated.

Petros Levounis, MD, MA
Director, The Addiction Institute of New York
Chief, Division of Addiction Psychiatry
The St. Luke's and Roosevelt Hospitals
Associate Clinical Professor of Psychiatry
Columbia University College of Physicians and Surgeons
New York, NY

PART ONE

The Basics

Is it normal for kids to try drugs?

How do I know if my child is using?
What behaviors should I look for?

Is there any simple way to ask my daughter
if she has a drug problem?

More . . .

1. Could my child actually be doing drugs?

Yes. Parents have exhibited different responses upon learning that their child has used drugs. This varies from disbelief, denial, surprise, and feelings of hurt and betrayal to stating that their suspicions have been confirmed. Recently, I had a male adolescent for evaluation whose legal guardian is his maternal aunt. His mother, who accompanied him for the meeting, was reacting indifferently to his drug use. At the same time, the mother acknowledged that her own bouts of drug abuse also contribute to why he is using. Whatever reason that may be, what is important is what you will have to do next.

2. Is it normal for kids to try drugs?

If you consider whether it is a norm or a passing phase for kids to try drugs, the answer is no. Most kids do not go through such a phase. Contrary to popular belief, up to 80% of adolescents transition to adulthood with minimal difficulties. Adolescence is when major decisions involving education, career, relationships, and lifestyle options are made, often with lifelong outcomes. The understanding of how substance use is embedded in the context of adolescent transition and identifying the context for its initiation and maintenance offers advantages for intervention. About 25% of adolescents who try drugs do not fare well, with many not receiving the help they need. It is rare that someone first uses illicit substances after he or she turns 20. In addition, the primary causes of drug-induced mortality and morbidity are preventable social, environmental, and social factors. It is more important to address the vulnerabilities that predispose adolescents to develop substance **use**. A number of adolescents are exposed to gateway drugs (see Question 11),

Use

Attempt at drug use that may not necessarily result in abuse or dependence.

but the majority of those adolescents who use drugs do not develop full-blown **addiction**. Only a subset of substance-using adolescents meets criteria for **abuse** or **dependence**. It is a diverse phenomenon involving different drug classes, patterns, and causes. The adolescents with difficulties have been on a deviant developmental trajectory since an early age marked by the presence of risk factors. For adolescents, there are clear-cut risk factors contributing to development of serious drug use. Despite the lifetime prevalence of substance use across all age groups and in both genders of approximately 30%, only 6% qualify for a lifetime diagnosis of abuse or dependence. Peak prevalence of substance abuse/dependence diagnosis is between 18 and 29 years of age. A report in 2006 affirmed that 6% of adolescents between ages 12 and 17 are deemed in need of substance abuse treatment.

Adolescents have responded in different ways about drug use. For marijuana, their justifications include, "It's not a drug"; "It's a plant"; "It's natural, like medicine"; I am not an addict"; "You don't get addicted to **weed**." Some have even mentioned that one is only addicted if one is not able to stop using it. It is not unlikely that marijuana is laced with other drugs like cocaine or heroin, and adolescents would know how they have reacted differently to these compared to marijuana alone.

3. What is the recent data on adolescent drug use?

The Office of National Drug Control Policy provided statistics showing a significant downturn in usage levels. An important source for this information is an annual representative survey sampling of American adolescents, college students, and adults through age fifty. Monitoring

THE BASICS

Addiction

Also known as dependence, addiction is a brain disease resulting from a chronic pattern of drug use characterized by compulsive engagement in drug seeking behaviors, with loss of sense of control, despite harmful consequences.

Abuse

Defined as addiction, although seen to have lesser criteria to meet the definition.

Dependence

A term that applies to addiction, involving drugs with either or both psychological dependence (perception of not being able to live or function without drugs) and physical dependence (tolerance and withdrawal).

Weed

Street name for marijuana.

the Future (MTF) has been conducted annually by the University of Michigan's Institute for Social Research since 1975. It is supported by the National Institute on Drug Abuse. In the most recent Monitoring the Future Study (2008), 19.6% of eighth graders, 34.1% of tenth graders, and 47.4% of twelfth graders reported using any illicit drug within their lifetimes.

Among the drugs that generally held steady in at least two of the three grades monitored were any illicit drug, marijuana, any illicit drug other than marijuana (except for a significant decline in tenth grade), inhalants, hallucinogens taken as a class (although twelfth graders showed a nonsignificant increase in 2007–2008), LSD, hallucinogens other than LSD, PCP, ecstasy (MDMA), sedatives (barbiturates), tranquilizers, heroin, narcotics other than heroin (data available for twelfth grade only), OxyContin, and Vicodin, specifically.

These youngsters also report fairly easy to very easy access to drugs. Accessibility was highest for marijuana at 90%, approaching beyond 95% for alcohol and 40% for opioids. Preventive measures should therefore begin even before the eighth grade.

4. How do I know if my child is using? What behaviors should I look for?

There is *no* certain way to know when your child is using. For the most part, a number of telltale signs add up, leading to parental knowledge. As our kids are in school, most of the troubling signs start with unaccounted tardiness, disinterest in school, not finishing schoolwork, and by being called by a school official recommending that your child be drug tested. You might not even think that your child's changes are due to drugs.

Parents have mentioned that their children started to hang out with kids known to use drugs. The old adage, "Tell me who your friends are and I will tell you who you are" reflects how your kids associate with those who may or may not be users. It is important to raise your suspicion for any change in behavior out of his/her usual ways and rule out drug effects as one of the causes.

When adolescents are **intoxicated** with cannabis (marijuana), behaviors include incessant laughing, withdrawal, irritability, acting suspiciously, and the more commonly reported glassy eyes. Your son may even spend less time with you to avoid being noticed. He may skip meals with the family and go straight to his room. There may also be changes in appetite. He may even sneak out at night to eat. Other changes in behavior can be odd, like keeping to himself; hearing voices; or being self-absorbed, paranoid, or extremely anxious. There maybe other signs, like empty bottles of alcohol that were intentionally hidden, cigarette butts, paper rolls, lighters, empty bags, leaf residues, or pipes. For parents who have been prescribed pain medications (in particular the opioid medications like acetaminophen and hydrocodone [Percocet or Vicodin]), missing supplies can raise suspicions.

It sometimes can be hard to even think that our kids are capable of doing drugs. Drug use should be considered as one of the possible causes of your child's behavior changes so that early intervention to avoid more serious consequences can be done.

It is important to raise your suspicion for any change in behavior out of his/her usual ways and rule out drug effects as one of the causes.

Intoxicated

More sophisticated term for being under the influence of drugs.

5. What is considered a drug? Alcohol? Caffeine? Marijuana? Herbal supplements/vitamins?

The term "drug" can generally be applied to a substance that falls into any of the following categories: medications prescribed by physicians to treat medical conditions, over-the-counter vitamin supplements and herbal plants requiring no doctor prescriptions, toxins that can have adverse or life threatening effects, and substances with potential for abuse. For our purpose, we are interested in substances with a potential for abuse because of their positive reinforcing effects with repeated use: we experienced something we like, which makes us use these drugs again and again. Some would not consider caffeine as a drug, but it is the most commonly used stimulant and is ingested by many people to produce alertness. A lot of people drink a cup of coffee or tea as part of their morning routine. With repeated use, you may experience headache, fatigue, drowsiness, or dysphoria if you skip your morning coffee, which are symptoms of withdrawal. Caffeine withdrawal is actually a diagnosable medical condition. Some individuals report that they have difficulty cutting down their use and inability to function without having that cup or series of cups during the course of the day. Caffeine dependence, however, is not yet considered a diagnosable condition.

Caffeine is the most commonly used stimulant and is ingested by many people to produce alertness.

6. I do not see any problems at all. Is there any chance that maybe my son is telling the truth when he says he's not using drugs?

It may be hard to ask kids if they are using. For the most part, even when you're frequently asking, they will continue to deny usage. To start, you might not notice anything out of the ordinary, but your neighbors or your son's school might have. As parents, you always want to give your son the benefit of the doubt. He might even accuse you of not trusting him. One helpful way to look at this is to support your concerns with evidence. Do not be lulled into complacency by a single drug test. Rather, random drug tests with negative results in addition to good performance in school, knowing who his friends are, good demeanor, and his continued involvement with his usual activities are more comforting than simply being verbally reassured by your son. It is not at all surprising that parents do not even know how to ask about their children's drug use. They might have an idea and nothing more their son or daughter is using or had used. It is important that you know for sure and learn what information to get.

7. Is there any simple way to ask my daughter if she has a drug problem?

For parents, an easy way to ask a child about drug usage is by using an easy to remember acronym, the CRAFFT screening method, composed of the following:

1. *Car*—Have you ever ridden in a car driven by someone (including yourself) who was "high" or had been using alcohol or drugs?
2. *Relax*—Do you use alcohol or drugs to relax, feel better about yourself, or fit in?
3. *Alone*—Do you ever use alcohol or drugs while alone?
4. *Forget*—Do you ever forget things you did while using alcohol or drugs?

5. *Friends or Family*—Do your family members or friends ever tell you that you should cut down on your drinking or drug use?

6. *Trouble*—Have you ever gotten into trouble while you were using alcohol or drugs?

If your son or daughter answers yes to two or more of these questions, he or she probably has a substance abuse problem.

Another way to assess your daughter's drug dependence is to fall back on the trust you have developed with her peers. This is especially true for friends who have stopped hanging out with your daughter because of her alleged use—they can give some clues about changes in your daughter's behavior.

Another screening questionnaire is the CAGE (cut down, annoyed, guilty, eye opener) questionnaire:

1. *Cut down*—Have you ever felt you needed to cut down on your drinking?

2. *Annoyed*—Have people annoyed you by criticizing your drinking?

3. *Guilty*—Have you ever felt guilty about drinking?

4. *Eye-opener*—Have you ever felt you needed a drink first thing in the morning (eye-opener) to steady your nerves or to get rid of a hangover?

8. Does drug use result from a defect in character?

We tend to separate inheritable (genetic) effects on one hand from environmental influences on the other. A more helpful and practical way is to determine how much of these influences play a role. Some kids can drink large quantities of alcohol and still be able to walk, and others become tipsy with just a drink or two. In the case of alcohol use disorders, genetic factors are thought to account for 60% of risk factors. A person's **level of response**, which is unique only to alcohol, is genetically determined by multiple genes. It measures how sensitive one is to alcohol, and one would tend to drink less if he or she is a high responder. Studies found that a low level of response in adolescents correlates with the current level of drinking and is predictive of alcohol use disorders later in life. Level of response interacts with factors such as peer influence, one's expectation of the effects of drinking, and stress. Especially with adolescents, peer influence is the most important factor outside of the home in determining continued use or maintenance of sobriety following treatment. Another study found that adolescents with low levels of response are more likely to have peers who drink more; these adolescents have poorer outcomes.

> **Level of response**
>
> A measure of one's sensitivity to alcohol. Someone with a low level of response would tend to consume more. It is unique to alcohol.

9. Is it okay if I want to keep my child's drug use a secret?

It is common for involved parents to want to keep their child's drug use a secret, perhaps even from their spouses, but it is not a good idea. During evaluations, parents are filled with shame, and more likely, with helplessness. Secrecy puts the parents further away from their support system when they most need it and makes it more difficult to help the youngster attain sobriety. Some parents still hope that the situation is not as bad as they think it is; they may ignore their kids and simply not do anything, or they may consider it a "phase" that will end. However, taking control and acknowledging some gaps in skills in dealing with drug use is taking the first step in healing.

Parents possibly lack the necessary support to start with. I have met with single parents, often mothers or even grandparents as primary caregivers, who feel isolated or even want to solve the problems on their own. Encouraging them to develop a support system is key in achieving and supporting their child's sobriety. A number of these supports can include the church, a close family member, a friend, and even a care provider.

Parents have expressed concern about not wanting their child's school to know that he or she is using for fear of being expelled from school. Enforcement of drug testing by schools is guided by policies with which parents should be familiar. With positive results, suspensions are coupled with mandatory awareness classes and probation, the length of which may be increased with subsequent reoffenses. Students are usually asked to receive counseling and complete treatment as a prerequisite to returning to school. Expulsion is reserved for after repeated recidivism. One of the discussions I have with parents is to establish that only relevant information can be shared with specific school personnel, and even then only *with* their consent. Federal and state laws are stringent about confidentiality issues regarding mental health treatment and substance abuse treatment. However, the school can also be used as an ally. Some schools have even placed substance abuse counselors on staff to specifically address this need.

10. What is self-medication?

There are certain situations where the primary reason that kids start smoking marijuana or using drugs is to make them feel better or as a means to cope—whether to forget family issues or school problems, or to treat depression, anxiety, or disordered thoughts; this is called

self-medication. I have heard some kids say they were using marijuana to "dampen the voices." It is not unlikely that adolescents resort to drugs to feel happier and to feel less alienated. Children who are traumatized, including those who have been physically, emotionally, and sexually abused, use drugs to numb themselves. They might say, "I don't want to feel anything," or "I do not want to remember it." Drugs can be abused specifically for their effects. Individuals who are depressed tend to use drugs with activating effects, such as cocaine. For those who try to avoid pain or anxiety, alcohol or opioids may be the drug of choice. I have also heard from people abusing heroin that "it just makes me feel nothing." Although drugs can in fact be helpful initially, usage will eventually take on a life of its own and become a problem itself. When that occurs, drug problems will be on top of the previous problem for which they were initially used. It is therefore very important to look at what originally motivated someone to use drugs. This is one of the goals of recovery. It is not uncommon that when adolescents have become sober, they disclose these traumatic issues. It is important that as parents, you are mindful of these possibilities.

11. What are gateway drugs?

Gateway drug is a term that resulted from studies of a segment of a population (epidemiological studies) linking earlier use of cigarettes, alcohol, and cannabis, followed by use of more serious drugs like cocaine, heroin, PCP, methamphetamine, etc. It is not fair to depict nicotine, alcohol, and cigarettes as less serious, as they *do* cause significant impairment in your child's functioning. In fact, early cigarette use is associated with later substance use more than half the time. Decreased perception of risk contributes to why kids start using, as more serious problems do not play

Self-medication
The use of drugs, especially the initial use of drugs, to help one cope with problems or in an attempt to treat anxiety, depression, or disordered thoughts.

Gateway drug
Drug such as cigarettes, alcohol, or cannabis that is used first, before one moves on to more serious drugs like cocaine, heroin, PCP, methamphetamine, etc.

It is not fair to depict nicotine, alcohol, and cigarettes as less serious, as they do cause significant impairment in your child's functioning.

out until later on. There is a subset of adolescents who, by virtue of the severity of their conduct problems, do start with drugs like cocaine. They are more likely to be involved with serious problems with the law and to start to develop behavior problems at an earlier age. One study suggested that early adolescent substance use prevention programs that focus initially on the gateway drugs may cause long-term prevention of amphetamine use.

12. Nobody gets addicted to marijuana, right?

On the contrary, yes, people do become addicted to marijuana although a number of individuals view cannabis use as a soft drug with no potential for adverse consequences. I have likewise heard from adolescents that "It is not a drug . . . it's a plant. It is natural. They should legalize it. It is used for pain." Adults whose primary drug of choice is marijuana are berated during treatment in intensive drug rehabilitation programs or therapeutic communities (TCs), more than those who have used alcohol, cocaine, or heroin. Some argue that marijuana should be legalized. This opinion, in addition to more potent marijuana and diminished perceived risks, contribute to increased rate of use. A 2007 report from the Substance Abuse and Mental Health Services Administration revealed an increase to 16% of adults seeking treatment for primary cannabis abuse, up from 12% in 1997. This shows how serious and chronic marijuana use has become. In a 2008 study by Hasin, cannabis withdrawal has been found to occur with clearly defined symptoms. The symptoms included two factors, one characterized by weakness, increased sleeping, and psychomotor retardation, and the second by anxiety, restlessness, depression, and insomnia (difficulty sleeping).

13. What are some street names for drugs?

Street names for drugs evolved as a means for covert communication. Law enforcers should be familiar with these ever-evolving terms to improve familiarity, surveillance, and arrests of drug abusers. Some are included below:

Street names for drugs evolved as a means for covert communication.

Club drugs: vitamin K, jet (ketamine, roofies [Rohypnol], goop GHB), E (MDMA, bumping up: Methylenedioxymethamphetamine (MDMA) combined with powder cocaine), nubs (peyote)

Cocaine: Carrie, Charlie, coke, snow, blow, barbs, basa, base, aspirin, aunt, Aunt Nora, nose candy, marching powder, banana (marijuana or cigarettes laced with cocaine), Bazooka (cocaine, combination of crack and marijuana), sheet rocking (crack and LSD)

Hallucinogens: acid, mellow yellow, 100's, 25's, battery acid, California sunshine (Lysergic acid diethylamide [LSD]); buttons, cactus (mescaline); Mexican mushrooms (Psilocybin)

Heroin: Big H, China white, Mexican brown, Smack, boy-girl (heroin mixed with cocaine), beast (heroin and LSD)

Cannabis: baby, babysitter, J, bud, blunt, purple haze, pop, sour D, L, Ari, candy sticks (marijuana cigarettes laced with powdered cocaine), atom bomb (marijuana mixed with heroin)

Steroids: juice, pumpers, weight trainers, Georgia home boy (GHB), Arnolds, stackers,

Inhalants: moon gas, air blast, snappers, whiteout (isobutyl nitrite), pearls (amyl nitrite), whippets (nitrous oxide)

Ritalin: Vitamin R

THE BASICS

PART TWO

Risk Factors

I have family members who have used drugs before but do not now. Can this play a role in my child's drug use?

I have a friend whose son has ADHD and is also receiving counseling for drug abuse. Was her son at a higher risk for substance abuse because of his ADHD?

Is there a relationship between bipolar disorder (manic-depressive illness) and drug abuse?

Are the reasons for starting to use drugs the same as those that one has for continuing drug use?

More . . .

14. What makes one end up as an abuser or dependent?

Fortunately, we know who is more likely to end up having significant drug problems. Oftentimes, drug users share the same vulnerabilities with other psychological or mental conditions, that exert varying degrees of influence. These include known risk factors including mood problems (risk for drug use is increased by two in individuals with major depression, seven times with bipolar disorder, three times with panic disorder, and five times with schizophrenia). As human beings, we experience the usual ups and downs as we deal with daily demands. Mood problems in these cases are severe depressive episodes that are medical illnesses that cause significant distress and a decrease in the child's functioning. In the case of the typical bipolar disorder, mood shifts are characterized by a manic episode, a depressive episode, or a combination of both. A manic episode is characterized by a persistent elevated or irritable mood *and* racing thoughts, increased energy, decreased need for sleep, and involvement in other high-risk behaviors like joyriding, leaving home at indiscriminate hours when safety issues are at hand, indiscriminate or unprotected sex or sex with multiple partners, or even use of drugs. In this case, it is important to separate conduct problems masquerading as a bipolar equivalent. Youngsters can also have atypical symptoms (mixed symptoms or variable symptom presentation over the course of the day or weeks). Adolescents with bipolar disorder can even have episodic anger outbursts that seem disproportionate to what may have triggered it. Duration of symptoms can be short-lived or in rapid cycles. Youngsters with behavior problems (oppositional defiant disorder, conduct disorder, and attention-deficit hyperactivity disorder) and learning difficulties are also at increased risk. Although it can be typical and expected of kids to be assertive, these psychiatric conditions go beyond the norm for their age. Defiant behaviors include talking back, arguing a lot, and being disrespectful and disobedient. In addition, severe conduct problems take the form of staying out late, not following curfew, running away, and other more serious behaviors that disregard the rights of others, such as stealing, trespassing, and robbery. In girls with severe conduct problems, conduct can take the form of vicious backbiting and gossiping. Other factors include peer pressure, family discord, and parental drug use. As peers are the single most important social group for youngsters outside of the home, they play a major role in how kids start and maintain their drug use.

High-risk individuals probably have risks with a biologic basis. These include difficulties in planning, attention problems, and problems with reasoning. These make it likely that adolescents will exhibit their anger in inappropriate ways.

15. How do you define/where do you draw the line between use, abuse, and dependency/addiction?

Drug use occurs when one has used drugs with no resultant established pattern of habitual use, adverse consequences, or signs of dependence. Abuse and dependence is generally seen on a continuum with more criteria fulfilled for a dependence diagnosis. One has to first establish the presence of dependence, which when fulfilled for a specific drug, overrides a diagnosis of abuse. Abuse and dependence share the presence of a compulsive pattern of drug use and loss of control over use with adverse consequences. Dependence is further characterized by

Abuse and dependence is generally seen on a continuum with more criteria fulfilled for a dependence diagnosis.

Psychological dependence

Loss of control (obsessive preoccupation) and the need to use a drug without the necessary physiologic change. It is manifested as craving or loss of sense of control over use.

the presence of either or both **psychological dependence** and physiologic dependence. Psychological dependence is established when one experiences craving and a perceived inability to function without using the drug. Physical dependence is characterized by the presence of signs and symptoms of withdrawal and/or tolerance. Tolerance is experienced after repeated drug use, when the amount of the drug being used does not effect the same high or the amount needs to be increased over time to achieve the same high. Withdrawal occurs when certain body reactions or symptoms, sometimes specific for a particular drug, are experienced after discontinuing use of the drug.

16. Does my child's temperament play a role in his drug abuse?

Temperament, already evident and stable during infancy and early childhood, is defined as aspects of one's personality that are inborn rather than learned. These are usually defined along observable behaviors. Children described as having a "difficult temperament" (being emotional, having difficulties with change, or being overly sensitive or finicky) are at higher risk. They in turn exhibit externalizing (like anger outbursts) and internalizing (like anxiety or depression) problems by middle childhood and adolescence.

Other challenges include reduced attention span, increased impulsivity, and irritability. These are conditions that are seen in kids with attention-deficit hyperactivity disorder (ADHD).

17. What are the family and environmental risk factors associated with adolescent drug use?

There are heritable traits as indicated by twin and adoptive studies. They include:

Peer Factors

1. Peer substance use
2. Peer attitudes about substance use
3. Greater orientation (attachment) to peers
4. Perception(s) of peer substance use/attitudes

Parent/Family Risk Factors

1. Parental substance use
2. Parent beliefs/attitudes about substance use
3. Lack of closeness/attachment with parents
4. Lack of parental involvement in child's life
5. Lack of appropriate supervision/discipline

18. I have family members who have used drugs before but do not now. Can this play a role in my child's drug use?

This confers risk but at the same time can be taken as an advantage. If your son or daughter has a good relationship with family members who previously abused drugs, the relatives can set their own negative experiences with drug use as examples from which the adolescent can learn. Sometimes, these family secrets can be hard to talk about, but with sensitivity and support, it can be openly discussed. Twin studies also point to 40–60% heritability for drug abuse and **alcoholism**. Sons of fathers with **Type II alcoholism** are at a ninefold risk of developing

Alcoholism

Alcohol addiction or dependence, where there is uncontrolled alcohol use with adverse consequences

Type II alcoholism

Type of alcoholism characterized by onset of alcoholism before age of 25, male gender, and aggression.

19

alcoholism. Type II alcoholics are characterized by onset of alcoholism before age of 25, male gender, and aggression associated with or without alcohol consumption. They are likely to get excitement from new experiences (high novelty seeking), be unfazed by risks (low harm avoidance), and not be motivated by rewards (low reward dependence). In addition, parental alcoholism also confers increased risk to other psychiatric conditions like ADHD, conduct disorder (CD) and overanxious disorder. Interestingly, individuals with similar risks who are using drugs are more likely to spend more time together than that which can be explained by chance alone. They attract each other!

Interestingly, individuals with similar risks and who are using drugs are more likely to spend more time together than that which can be explained by chance alone. They attract each other!

19. Should I look for other conditions in addition to drug problems?

There are studies that track how often psychiatric conditions exist and what conditions usually go together. One study reported that 15–24-year-olds had the highest 12-month prevalence of any disorder, including substance abuse. Substance-abusing adolescents reveal high rates of coexisting mood disorders and behavior problems (conduct disorder). In a survey of adolescents in the community who abuse drugs, they are more likely to also suffer from mood problems. Individuals with severe problems with the law (such as those with antisocial personality disorder) have high rates of substance abuse. For adolescents with severe conduct problems and drug use, depression imparts risk far more severe than drug use alone. These adolescents abuse more drugs in combination, tend to have behavioral problems at an earlier age, and have increased anxiety and attentional problems. Adolescents with history of PTSD were found to have increased risk for cannabis use *separate* from the effects of deviant peers, genetics, race, male gender, socioeconomic status, or having a substance-abusing parent. Therefore, the significant interaction of these problems indicates that these conditions warrant very aggressive treatment.

20. I have a friend whose son has ADHD and is also receiving counseling for drug abuse. Was her son at a higher risk for substance abuse because of his ADHD?

The combination of ADHD and CD appears to be a more robust risk factor for later substance abuse than CD alone. Parents of children with CD alone have lower rates of alcohol and drug abuse than the parents of the conduct plus ADHD group. The parents in both of these groups had higher rates of children with substance abuse than the parents of children with ADHD alone. ADHD is found to occur in 30–50% of patients with co-occurring CD. ADHD was also shown to be associated with early onset of cigarette smoking. In addition, mood/anxiety disorders and conduct disorders, which are elevated in smokers, are also associated with ADHD. These conditions go along with each other to some extent.

21. Is there a relationship between bipolar disorder (manic–depressive illness) and drug abuse?

Adolescent-onset bipolar disorder is associated with higher risk for drug use compared to childhood-onset bipolar disorder. In fact, it ranks just slightly lower than conduct disorder (CD) in conferring that risk. When these two co-occur, recovery is more difficult, and both have to be treated aggressively.

22. Do drugs cause problems with anger?

Drug use increases the risk for adolescents to get involved in fights. In some ways, drugs offer a reason for adolescents to act on their anger. Some get disinhibited by drug use. You might have heard a story about a youngster known to be meek and quiet who then becomes violent while under the influence of drugs. It is also likely that drug use is intertwined with antisocial behavior where anger is channeled through gang activities ("jumping" other kids). On the other hand, some kids avoid acting on their anger and using drugs as a means to regain control or even numb their feelings. The use of drugs can also act as a way to deal with pent-up anger resulting from family problems, school problems, or even from boyfriend/girlfriend issues. Irritability and aggression can be identified as behaviors for which medications are prescribed, especially if anger impedes benefits from psychosocial interventions.

Individuals who act on their anger are at increased risk for later substance abuse. A derived scale, the Violence Proneness Scale (VPS) from the Drug Use Screening Inventory (DUSI-R, see Question 57 for more information on this), is significantly predictive of aggressive behavior in young boys five to seven years later. The VPS established with 82% accuracy which male youths tested at age 16 did and did not give drugs in exchange for sex three years later. The VPS can be a very useful psycho-educational tool for parents during initial evaluations in identifying and discussing future risks especially if no treatment is provided.

23. There is a high rate of alcoholism in my family, so my child must be doomed to develop this condition, right?

This is a fatalistic sentiment expressed by parents every now and then. While there is a strong heritability for drug use, especially for alcohol use (up to 60%), this is still seen only as a vulnerability: no complete causal relationship has emerged from studies. There are things that can be done before problems start. Your child can benefit from getting involved with extracurricular activities or sports. Spending quality time with your child as a family will be important in his or her upbringing. As parents, you can set living examples of leading a sober life. It takes courage to even talk about the presence of this risk factor in your family. Doing so affords a more open, honest, and candid conversation so that other, healthier choices can be made. His or her keeping sober friends that you also know decreases this risk. This will require your commitment, time, and effort as you and your child get involved with help.

24. Putting risks aside, are there any factors that can protect my child from substance abuse?

We know that certain factors have a greater chance of protecting children from using drugs—female gender; higher socioeconomic status; high academic aspiration or achievement; close and affectionate relationships with parents or family members; and absence of parental marital problems, chronic conflict, or alcohol abuse. In addition, family's involvement with church confers protection. Church activities allow for the youngster's involvement in activities promoting social interaction with peers, moral development, and appropriate self-control. Treatment of co-occurring psychiatric conditions also decreases risk of future drug problems. It is therefore imperative that general difficulties observed early on in childhood be discussed with your primary doctors or pediatrician to establish need for further evaluation/referral and early treatment.

25. Are there other characteristics that are likely to contribute to increased drug or alcohol use?

A risk profile was developed in a study to predict those who intended to use alcohol and those who did not among fifth and sixth graders. Rejection of parental authority was correlated with sixth graders more than with fifth graders. This is suggestive of a dwarfing importance of family role as adolescents get older and peer pressure becomes a more predominant factor. This is why parents should rely on really knowing who their children's friends are. It may be helpful to invite your children's friends to your home as a means to know them and to get acquainted with their parents for networking. Try to avoid criticizing your child's friends. Acknowledge that these friends are an increasingly important part of your child's support system as he or she tries to define his or her own identity. Realize that your child also balances peer pressure as you encourage him or her to develop independent thinking. Work with your child in playing out the consequences of choices so that he or she may avoid grave mistakes.

P300 is brain surface electrical activity that is most strongly picked up in the parietal lobes. It is measured by an electroencephalogram (EEG), which is a procedure for which electrodes are attached at different parts of the scalp. P300 is involved in evaluating situations and decision-making processes. A blunted P300 is associated in adolescents with alcohol use and is found to be highly heritable. Its effects are found independent of the adverse effects of alcohol use.

26. Are the reasons for starting to use drugs the same as those that one has for continuing drug use?

No. A number of reasons identified by kids to begin using drugs include curiosity, as a means to kill time or relax, or being pressured by friends, saying "My friends try it, so why shouldn't I?" or "It's cool with my friends." Some kids deny the seriousness of trying drugs, saying, "It's not a drug" or "I won't get addicted to it." This might progress to repeated use because of the drugs' positive reinforcing effects (feeling good when **high**). A number of adolescents talk about the sense of belongingness that comes about when using drugs with friends and that this boosts their self esteem and morale. Continued use is again tied up with diminished perception of risk or harm and the fact that serious aftermath is not experienced until later on (adverse consequences are delayed). In cases of opioids (morphine or pains medications like Percocet [acetaminophen with oxycodone], codeine, or Tylenol 3 [acetaminophen and codeine]), one important reason for continuing to use drugs is to avoid uncomfortable **withdrawal** effects upon discontinuation of the drug.

High

Street term for being under the influence of drugs.

Withdrawal

Uncomfortable or even painful bodily complaints and signs that exist after drug use is stopped. Occurs with dependence.

PART THREE

Alcohol Abuse in Adolescents

What is binge drinking?

What signs and symptoms should I look for to recognize alcohol poisoning? What should I do if I suspect my son of alcohol poisoning?

What preventive measures are effective to deal with underage drinking?

More . . .

27. I often hear about adolescents who get alcohol poisoning because they drink too much at once. Is this a common occurrence?

I have encountered a number of adolescents (females outnumbering males) who are referred through the emergency rooms for **alcohol poisoning**. This results from significant amounts of alcohol ingested in a short period of time by individuals who have not been regular drinkers. The adolescents that I have worked with reported using hard liquors like Hennesey, Bacardi, E and J, and Smirnoff. Compared to beer volume by volume, hard liquors require smaller amounts to achieve similar alcohol levels and therefore take less time to achieve toxic levels. Kids are also unable to pace their consumption.

Alcohol poisoning

Results from consuming large amounts of alcohol in a short period of time. Binge drinking is the most common cause and results in ineffective breathing and impaired blood circulation. This is a medical emergency where 911 calls have to be made.

There are very few published studies, and even fewer involving Americans, that establish how common alcohol poisoning is. A European study (Kuzelova et al., 2009) looked at alcohol intoxication that required hospital admissions in children and adolescents. Covering a nine-year period, this study found that the average age of presentation is 15, and the number of children requiring admissions increased every year. The average alcohol concentration was 1.98 ± 0.57 g/L, and this level increased in the last four years compared to the previous four years.. The severity of poisoning also increased in relation to blood alcohol levels.

Alcohol levels go beyond the legal limit of intoxication, which, depending on the state, ranges from 0.1 to 0.15 mg/dL. They had no recollection of events and had blacked out. A number of them had to be treated in intensive care units. A few of them also ingested other psychoactive agents like marijuana, which can be laced with cocaine, PCP, or embalming fluids. A few have disclosed using downers (benzodiazepines like diazepam, Xanax [alprazolam], or Ativan [lorazepam]), which can significantly increase depressant effects when used with alcohol. Some of these individuals ended up losing their lives from significant respiratory depression or infection of the lungs due to aspiration related to decreased responsiveness.

28. What is the alcohol equivalent to one drink?

One drink is equal to 12 g of ethanol, which is equal to 1.5 oz. of 80-proof liquor (40% ethanol) such as whiskey or gin, 12 oz. of regular beer (7.2 proof, 3.6% ethanol in the United States). Just one drink increases blood alcohol level of a 150-pound individual by 15–20 mg/dL. The body clears one drink in an hour at 20 mg/dL. Most (90%) of the alcohol is excreted through the liver by the enzyme alcohol dehydrogenase to acetaldehyde. This is then broken down to acetic acid and carbon dioxide (CO_2) by acetaldehyde dehydrogenase.

29. What is an acceptable pattern of drinking?

There is no acceptable pattern for adolescents. Moderate drinking by adults is acceptable. In adults, population studies point to the following as moderate drinking: up to two drinks in a day for males and up to one drink a day for females, and *not* as an average over several days. Every now and then, I encounter adolescents who report early drinking, as introduced by family members during dinners or by alcohol-using relatives. It may also be cultural. In a study by Mayzer and Zucker, **early first drinking (EFD)**, defined as the first drink by 12 to 14 years of age, was associated with more delinquent behaviors than aggression. EFD was also disproportionately likely at both 3–5 and 12–14 years of age in children with high delinquent behaviors and was uncommon in those with low levels of delinquency. Alcohol consumption among young adults will continue to be an issue. In the United States, a minimum of 21 years old is the legal requirement in all states for alcohol consumption. There are about 10.8 million underage drinkers in the United States.

30. What is binge drinking?

Binge drinking is defined as the consumption of five or more drinks in a row for boys and four or more in a row for girls. Males are twice as likely to binge as females. Most people who binge drink are not alcohol dependent. Even for adults, approximately 92% of those who drink excessively report binge drinking in the month prior. Most (75%) binge drinking episodes involve adults over age 25 years. Binge drinkers are 14 times more likely to report alcohol-impaired driving than nonbinge drinkers.

About 90% of the alcohol consumed by youth under the age of 21 years in the United States is in the form of binge drinking. The proportion of current drinkers who binge is highest in the 18–20-year-old group. Binge drinking begins around age 13, tends to increase during adolescence, and peaks in young adulthood (ages 18–22). Binge drinking during the past 30 days was reported by 8% of youth aged 12–17 and 30% of those aged 18–20.

Among persons under the legal drinking age (12–20), 15% were binge drinkers and 7% were heavy drinkers. Individuals who are drunk are more likely to drive after drinking, ride with drivers who have been drinking, not wear seat belts, carry weapons, get involved in physical fights, engage in unplanned/unprotected sex, and use illicit drugs.

31. What is the level of alcohol that is dangerous?

The effects of alcohol have differing degrees of danger. One's blood alcohol level (BAL) or blood alcohol content (BAC) should be an indicator of whether one is in danger from the alcohol itself or whether one might engage in dangerous behavior or be prone to having or causing an accident of some sort. The following list shows the different bodily experiences at increasing blood alcohol levels:

- **0.02–0.03 BAC**: Slight euphoria and loss of shyness; coordination is maintained.
- **0.04–0.06 BAC**: Feeling of well-being, relaxation, lowered inhibitions, sensation of warmth, euphoria, minor impairment of reasoning and memory.
- **0.07–0.09 BAC**: Slight impairment of balance, speech, vision, reaction time, and hearing; euphoria; reduced judgment and self-control. One with a BAC of 0.08 is legally impaired and for a number of states, it is illegal to drive at this level. You will probably believe that you are functioning better than you really are.
- **0.10–0.125 BAC**: Severe motor incoordination, slurred speech, hearing and vision are impaired, euphoria. The BAC at which it is illegal to drive in West Virginia and Ohio is 0.10.

- **0.13–0.15 BAC**: Gross motor impairment and lack of physical control, blurred vision and loss of balance, anxiety and restlessness, severely impaired judgment and perception.
- **0.16–0.19 BAC**: Uncomfortable mood predominates; nausea may appear. The drinker has the appearance of a sloppy drunk.
- **0.20 BAC**: Disorientation. Assistance needed to stand or walk, possible inability to elicit pain if injured. Nausea and vomiting, possible choking with vomiting. Blackouts.
- **0.25 BAC**: All mental, physical, and sensory functions are severely impaired. Increased risk of asphyxiation from choking on vomitus and of serious risk of aspiration.
- **0.30 BAC**: Stupor, disorientation.
- **0.35 BAC**: Possibility of coma. This is the level of surgical anesthesia.
- **0.40 BAC and higher**: Onset of coma and possible death due to respiratory arrest.

I have treated adults who are able to carry a conversation and do not appear intoxicated even at a level of 0.25. This shows an extreme level of **tolerance** to alcohol.

Tolerance

A condition that is marked by the need for an increased amount of the drug abused to achieve the same high or attenuated reinforcing effects at the same amount. Occurs with drug dependence.

Alcohol poisoning is a medical emergency and 911 should be called immediately.

32. What signs and symptoms should I look for to recognize alcohol poisoning? What should I do if I suspect my son of alcohol poisoning?

Alcohol poisoning is a medical emergency and 911 should be called immediately. Symptoms of alcohol poisoning include alcohol on one's breath; slow or irregular breathing (less than 8 breaths a minute or 10 or more seconds between breaths); cold, clammy, pale, or bluish skin (a sign that not enough oxygen is provided); unconsciousness; and vomiting. It is very important that the airways are unobstructed; you may need to position your son on his side to avoid aspiration of vomitus. You may even have to support his breathing by mouth-to-mouth resuscitation.

33. I heard about the Amethyst Initiative. What is it?

College presidents from about 135 of the nation's best-known universities, including Duke, Dartmouth, and Ohio State, have called on lawmakers to consider lowering the drinking age from 21 to 18, saying current laws actually encourage dangerous binge drinking on campus. This was spearheaded by John McCardell, President Emeritus of Middlebury College, who questioned the 1984 federal highway law that financially penalizes states with a drinking age below 21. Amethyst came from the Greek words "a" (not) and "methustos" (intoxicated). Mythology states that Amethyst, a young girl, angered the god Dionysius after she got intoxicated with alcohol. She sought the help of Diana, who turned her into a white stone. After learning this, Dionysius felt sad and tears fell into his wine cup, which spilled onto the white stone and turned it purple. Amethyst is seen as an antidote against intoxication. The Web site (www.amethystinitiative.org) talks about amethyst being an appropriate symbol for this initiative, "which aims to encourage moderation and responsibility as an alternative to the drunkenness and reckless decisions about alcohol that mark the experience of many young Americans."

In New Jersey, hearings were conducted to address this issue with Mothers Against Drunk Driving (MADD), and the directors of the state's Division of Highway Traffic Safety and of Alcohol Beverage Control testified that legal drinking age laws saved lives. Since the drinking age was raised to 21 in New Jersey in the 1980s, there has been a 78% decrease in the number of 18- to 20-year-olds killed in drunken-driving crashes. This is solid evidence that the higher age requirement is, in fact, helping to prevent such accidents.

34. What preventive measures are effective to deal with underage drinking?

There are public policies that have been effective, including:

1. Increasing price of alcohol
2. Increasing minimum age to purchase
3. Restricting access for retail alcohol sale
4. Regulating density or concentration of retail outlets
5. Regulating types of retail outlets
6. Restriction of licenses of retail outlets
7. Restricting service of alcohol (IDs)
8. Enforcing drinking and driving laws (random breath testing)
9. Setting BAC limits for drunk driving (0.05%–0.08%; for young drivers: 0.00%–0.02%, **zero tolerance**)
10. Implementing administrative license revocation laws
11. Implementing graduated driving licenses

Zero tolerance

A requirement that one's blood alcohol level be 0%.

12. Using automobile ignition interlocks
13. Restricting advertising
14. Placing warning labels on beverages
15. Implementing keg registration
16. Community interventions

Practices with solid evidence include:

1. Increasing retail price of alcohol
2. Increasing minimum drinking age
3. Restricting hours and days of alcohol use
4. Zero tolerance policies for driving while under the influence of alcohol
5. Establishing limits on the retail sale of alcohol
6. Establishing lower BAC limits for driving

PART FOUR

Steroid Use in Adolescents

My son is into sports at school. What type of drugs might he encounter as an athlete?

What is the usual dosage and period of time for which steroids are administered?

What are the telltale signs of steroid abuse?

More . . .

35. My son is into sports at school. What type of drugs might he encounter as an athlete?

As athletes are driven to win, with no room for failure, they are more likely to seek performance-enhancing substances. Male student athletes were at a high risk for heavy alcohol use and steroids as they deal with more stress in meeting the demands of both roles. When taken for a period of 10–20 weeks, a high dose of steroids can increase lean body mass, size, and strength, with or without exercise. Most notably, however, are steroids' performance-enhancing effects if combined with a training regimen and a high-caloric and high-protein diet. Anabolic-androgenic steroids (AASs) produce heightened mood and decreased fatigue, prolonging physical exertion.

A study (Buckley et al., 1998) found that 6.6% of male high school seniors had tried steroids, with 67% onset of use by age 16, and 40% using multiple cycles. The Monitoring of the Future Study (2008) indicated that 1.4% of eighth graders, 1.4% of tenth graders, and 2.2% of twelfth graders have reported trying steroids at least once in their lifetime. Anabolic steroids are used primarily by males. Annual prevalence rates were 1.2%, 1.4%, and 2.5% for boys in grades 8, 10, and 12, compared with 0.5%, 0.5%, and 0.4% for girls, respectively.

A high level of steroid abuse has been exposed among professional athletes. A number of professional baseball players have been implicated or have disclosed using banned steroids during their careers. Serving as role models, these athletes may well have contributed to adolescents' decrease in perceived risks of use. The nonmedical use of AASs has been banned by a number of organizations including the International Olympic Committee, the

U.S. Olympic Committee, and the National Collegiate Athletic Association. A number of medical associations have likewise denounced their nonmedical use.

AASs have multiple medical uses; they have been used in trauma, extensive surgery, and growth and puberty delays. They also are used for AIDS-associated wasting syndrome. Steroids reverse further breakdown in burns. They also show promising results in muscle wasting for patients with advanced kidney problems.

36. What is the usual dosage and period of time for which steroids are administered?

For their performance-enhancing effects, testosterone preparations are usually given by injection at doses of 25–200 mg weekly. Doses are abused to as much as three times the recommended use. Steroids taken by mouth range from 35 to 200 mg weekly and are abused up to four times the recommended dose. Usually, injection and oral forms are used during a 6–12-week cycle. Injectable preparations are less likely to cause liver problems. Oral forms are cleared from the body faster and are preferred to avoid detection. **Stacking** is when multiple steroids are used at the same time. **Pyramiding** is when doses are increased through a cycle allowing for doses to be increased 10–40 times the usual dose. These two methods decrease the side effects of steroids. It is common that individuals also take supplements (vitamins, creatine, and other protein supplements) to boost the steroid effects. Others also use other medications like tamoxifen, a cancer medication, to reduce risk of breast enlargement. Sources often include gyms, which procure them illegally (via foreign mail orders and the Internet). Quality or even whether these are actual steroids cannot be ensured.

Injectable preparations are less likely to cause liver problems.

Stacking

The use of multiple steroids at the same time.

Pyramiding

Increasing doses of steroids through a cycle allowing for doses to be increased 10–40 times the usual dose.

37. What are the telltale signs of steroid abuse?

Telltale signs include yellowish discoloration of the skin, high blood pressure, decrease in testicle size, change in voice pitch, breast enlargement, which can be permanent after long-term use, tendon fractures, stopping of growth, severe acne, baldness, abscesses from needle punctures, and pinkish to silver streaks on the skin. Steroids also cause increases in positive mood (mania) or depression, violence, or disordered thinking. The physical examination clearance from physicians, who must have increased awareness of the problem, provides the time to note any changes that can be attributed to AAS abuse.

There are no clear-cut profiles that separate those who abuse steroids from others. Sports requiring strength and power (football, wrestling, and track) are most closely associated with AAS. Other adolescents look to steroids to help attain what is in their eyes a more attractive body.

38. What can parents do to prevent their son or daughter from becoming involved in steroid abuse?

Educational programs that take place before use starts have been suggested to be more effective over drug testing policies. Discussion as part of providing information has to be balanced and should both cover the desired effects and side effects. Supervised training programs are also key. Steroids do not play any legitimate role in sports. Period.

Steroids do not play any legitimate role in sports. Period.

PART FIVE

Drug Abuse

I heard that my son took his classmate's Adderall.
Should I be concerned?

Why does prescription drug abuse seem
to be such a problem nowadays?

My friend's daughter was seen huffing something
at home. Should my friend be worried?

What are the effects and dangers of club drugs?

More . . .

39. I heard that my son took his classmate's Adderall. Should I be concerned?

Stimulant

Class of medications that is the first line of treatment for ADHD and is not complicated by drug use.

Yes. Adderall (dextroamphetamine salts) is a **stimulant** medication medically approved for ADHD. It can also improve memory and wakefulness in healthy individuals, which makes it a drug of choice during exam preparations. Side effects are the extension of its intended benefits and are dose dependent. These effects include euphoria, agitation, hyperthermia (dysregulated increase in body temperature), seizures, hearing voices, and suspiciousness (paranoia). Some individuals combine opioids (**downers**) like heroin with stimulants (Ritalin [methylphenidate] or Adderall) to counteract the high. **Overdoses** can lead to heart rhythm abnormalities, heart attack, and breakdown of muscle, leading to kidney shutdown, status epileptics, and brain hemorrhages.

Downers

Drugs whose primary effect is to induce motor slowing and sedation.

Overdose

Taking more than what is prescribed or suggested for a medication. It can be intentional or accidental.

40. My friend gave her Xanax to her daughter to help with her anxiety. Is this safe?

Short-acting

A brief duration of medication/drug effects, usually inversely related to how long it takes for the body to get rid of it.

No. Xanax (alprazolam) is a potent, **short-acting** benzodiazepine, which is primarily indicated for anxiety problems (used in severe panic disorder where individuals are not even able to leave their homes to get counseling). Compared to older medications like barbiturates (phenobarbital or Fioricet [a combination of butalbital and acetaminophen that is used for migraines]), benzodiazepines have less potential for abuse, but nevertheless are still addictive. They cause drowsiness, cross-eye, hypothermia, respiratory depression, stupor, and coma. The shorter acting and more potent these medications are, the more likely that they will cause dependence. Xanax is therefore more addictive than Klonopin (clonazepam) or Valium (diazepam) because it is relatively more potent and stays in the body the shortest time (has the shortest half-life). Five milligrams of diazepam is equivalent to 0.25 mg of alprazolam and is equivalent to 1 mg of clonazepam.

41. Why does prescription drug abuse seem to be such a problem nowadays?

Because there are so few studies, no definitive answers have been offered to explain the increased prevalence of adolescent prescription pain relievers (PPRs). In one study (Wu et al., 2008), increased PPR is seen in adolescents with depression or alcohol problems. A number of these adolescents would be missed if strict *DSM-IV* criteria for abuse or dependence are applied; they nevertheless exhibit impairments. Compared to adolescents with no *DSM-IV* symptoms, abusers are likely to be younger and not attending school, be in counseling, have impaired physical health, and have developed a major depressive episode. A reason offered for drug use is the relief of psychic or physical pain, as opposed to getting high.

In 2005, 1.4 million visits to the emergency room involved substance abuse, 37% of which were for prescription drug abuse. Their abuse is implicated in suicide attempts, 45% of which involved prescription medication and 56% of which involved sedatives and stimulants. Use of a **controlled substance** for reasons other than that for which it is prescribed, often in doses different than prescribed, results in disability and dysfunction. This is often in the context of illegal activity, aberrant medication-seeking behavior, and risk of harm to the abuser. Teens often use their parents' or their grandparents' pain medications, which are easily accessed from medicine cabinets. Remember the epidemic of OxyContin use? The long-term preparation

Teens often use their parents' or their grandparents' pain medications.

Controlled substance

Substances defined by the Drug Enforcement Agency with varying levels of addictive potential (based on schedules) and medicinal value.

capsule, when crushed, caused an immediate rush, which can cause severe intoxication and loss of breathing control, making it fatal to some individuals.

The most common way to obtain medication is from friends or family. (Beware the medicine cabinet!) Other common methods include obtaining medication from a physician, **physician hopping**, purchasing medication, or theft, usually from friends or relatives.

Physician hopping

A form of drug seeking behavior in which an individual sees multiple doctors to obtain the desired drug of abuse.

42. Who is more likely to abuse prescription drugs?

There are certain individuals who are more likely to misuse prescription drugs. Schepis and Sarin (2008) found the following characteristics: past year history of alcohol, nicotine, cannabis and cocaine or inhalant use; and past history of major depression. Sex differences were found, predominantly for opioids; females are more likely to steal medication or obtain it for free, whereas males are more likely to purchase medication or acquire it from a physician. White adolescents are more likely to buy opioids, whereas African American adolescents are more likely to misuse opioids obtained from a physician. Across medication classes, adolescents who recently acquired medication by purchasing it have the worst risk profile in terms of concurrent substance use and severity of prescription misuse. While opioid withdrawal is relatively benign, drug overdose can be fatal.

Although heroin is an illegal drug, it is worth mentioning here. A number of adults that I treated started abusing prescription opioids when they were younger to treat pain conditions. This pain can result from common things such as a tooth extraction or an injury that results in fractures and back pain. They would then use prescribed opioids more than intended and engage in aberrant drug-seeking behaviors, eventually moving to using street opioids, such as heroin.

Heroin is a highly addictive drug and is the most widely abused and rapidly acting of the opiates. It is derived from morphine, a naturally occurring substance from the poppy plant. Pure heroin is a white powder with a bitter taste and is rarely sold on the streets. Color differences are due to impurities. Another form of heroin, **black tar** heroin, is primarily available in the western and southwestern United States, with its color varying from dark brown to black. Heroin can be injected, smoked, or snorted, and injection is the most efficient way to administer low-purity heroin. Heroin can also be introduced through the skin, known as **popping**.

Black tar

A form of heroin that is primarily available in the western and southwestern United States, with its color varying from dark brown to black.

Popping

Introducing heroin into the top layers of the skin.

43. What are scheduled drugs?

The Drug Enforcement Administration (DEA), a federal arm of the Department of Justice, has issued guidelines and classification of drugs with addictive potential (see **Table 1**). Prescription and dispensing practices are governed by regulations, and violations result in penalties.

In some states, stimulant medications prescribed for ADHD are written in triplicate forms and can only be given monthly. The original prescription is given to the patient, one is kept by the physician for his or her records, and the other is kept by the pharmacy for record keeping.

This aims to encourage appropriate medication monitoring and avoid misuse and diversion. In New York, although benzodiazepines are classified as Schedule IV drugs, they are also written in triplicate forms to discourage misuse and diversion.

Physicians are given licenses to prescribe controlled substances; the license comes with a DEA number, without which no controlled medications can be prescribed. In New Jersey, there is an additional license number, the controlled drug substance number, that has to be renewed by physicians annually to prescribe these medications.

The DEA has allowed physicians to electronically prescribe stimulants, which allows the patients better access to their medication and still offers physicians the ability to monitor use of the medications.

Table 1 Schedules

Schedule	Restriction	Examples
I. No approved medical use	Illicit, cannot be prescribed	Heroin, phencyclidine (PCP), lysergic (LSD)
II. High abuse	No refills, no verbal orders from physicians, triplicates	Morphine, oxycodone, meth-amphetamine, secobarbital
III. Moderate	Max 5 refills/6 mo; verbal orders from physicians allowed in some states	Hydrocodone with acetaminophen
IV. Low to moderate	Max 5 refills/6 mo; verbal orders from physicians allowed	Benzodiazepines like Ativan (lorazepam), Xanax (alprazo-lam), Klonopin (clonazepam)
V. Limited abuse	May be over-the-counter (OTC) in some states	Diphenoxylate, dextrometorphan

Modified from http://www.justice.gov/dea/pubs/scheduling.html

44. What is methamphetamine, and what are its effects?

Methamphetamines are highly addictive central nervous system stimulants that can be injected, snorted, smoked, or orally ingested. Methamphetamine users feel a short yet intense rush when the drug is initially administered. The immediate effects of methamphetamine include increased activity and decreased appetite. Most methamphetamines distributed to the black market are produced in fly-by-night laboratories, which are sometimes even found in households. The ease of production and significant profits obtained from selling methamphetamine resulted in increased availability of illicit supply in the United States.

Of particular concern is how pseudoephedrine, a drug commonly found in cough and cold medicines, has been used to illegally manufacture methamphetamines. Requiring that this otherwise safe and effective over-the-counter (OTC) medication be available only by prescription may make it difficult to access for those who use it for its intended purposes. One way to reduce product misuse while also allowing access to the drug for consumers is to maintain the lowest effective dose in OTC preparations, which is 10 mg for pseudophedrine, and to restrict the maximum amount allowed for a single purchase.

45. What happens when someone abuses cough preparations?

Dextromethorphan (DMX) is a cough suppressant found in a variety of over-the-counter cold and cough medications. Like PCP (see Question 50) and ketamine (see Question 48), dextromethorphan is a

Dissociative anesthetic

Drugs primarily used in surgical operations whose effects can include hallucinations.

dissociative anesthetic, meaning its effects can include hallucinations. These preparations are available without prescriptions. Psychological effects depend on the amount ingested. Symptoms of abuse include confusion, dizziness, double or blurred vision, slurred speech, impaired physical coordination, abdominal pain, nausea and vomiting, rapid heartbeat, drowsiness, numbness of fingers and toes, and disorientation. Some users even experience plateaus ranging from mild distortions of color and sound to visual hallucinations and out-of-body, dissociative sensations and loss of motor control. I have treated a number of male adolescents with these problems; some have ingested as much as 240 mg daily. They have obtained DMX by shoplifting from drugstores. Serotonin is decreased by chronic abuse. Addicts needed antidepressant treatment due to prominent depressive symptoms resulting from low serotonin levels. In addition to drug use, two of these youngsters also suffered from ADHD. They eventually ended up in longer term residential treatment programs.

46. My friend's daughter was seen huffing something at home. Should my friend be worried?

Definitely. Inhalants include solvents (such as varnish), glues, adhesives, aerosol propellants (cleaning fluid, spray paint, and correction fluid), paint thinners, and fuels (gasoline, kerosene, and lighter fluid). Symptoms of intoxication include dizziness, incoordination, unsteady gait, involuntary movement of the eyes, slurred speech, lethargy, psychomotor retardation, generalized muscle weakness, tremors, blurred vision, double vision that could be as severe as disorientation, stupor, or coma. These drugs can easily be accessed and are of low cost, making them ideal for abuse. They are very toxic, can affect the white matter (supportive tissues) part of the brain, and can result in irreversible damage manifested as lasting motor incoordination, memory impairment, and forgetfulness.

47. What are the effects and dangers of club drugs?

Club drugs are a diverse group of psychoactive compounds that tend to be abused by teens and young adults at a nightclub, bar, rave, or trance scene. Raves are dance gatherings that continue for hours with repetitive and monotonous music where a cocktail of pills are given. Due to prolonged dancing and altered consciousness, individuals suffer from dehydration from lack of fluid intake. Gamma hydroxybutyrate (GHB), Rohypnol (flunitrazepam), ketamine, MDMA (ecstasy), and methamphetamines are some of the drugs in this group. MDMA is a synthetic drug similar to methamphetamine and the hallucinogen mescaline. Rohypnol and GHB have been used as **date rape drugs** as they sedate unsuspecting victims. GHB, available in an odorless, colorless liquid form or as a white powder material, is taken orally and is frequently combined with alcohol. This increases the risk of unintentional overdose which can result in respiratory depression. In addition to being used to incapacitate individuals for the commission of sexual assault/rape, GHB is also sometimes used by bodybuilders for its alleged anabolic effects. Xyrem (sodium oxybate), a product that contains GHB, is an approved prescription drug for narcolepsy, a medical condition characterized by excessive sleepiness. Xyrem is also prescribed for cataplexy, which is a medical condition characterized by the sudden loss of muscle tone usually in response to extreme

Club drugs

A diverse group of psychoactive compounds that tend to be abused by teens and young adults at a nightclub, bar, rave, or trance scene.

Date rape drugs

Drugs used to sedate unsuspecting victims for purposes of sexual advances.

of emotions. A commonly experienced form of cataplexy is falling down with bouts of laughter or anger. Whereas GHB is a schedule I drug, Xyrem is a schedule II drug; however, diversion is subject to schedule I penalties.

GHB is hard to detect because it is not routinely tested for during drug screens. The Project GHB Web site (http://www.projectghb.org) has extensive information on this subject and has also identified a number of support groups and a list of providers who can offer treatment and counseling.

48. What happens if humans use drugs meant for animals?

Ketamine, a tranquilizer used in animals, became popular in the 1980s. It is similar to reactions induced by PCP (see Question 50), such as dreamlike states and hallucinations. Ketamine is used to lace marijuana, and youngsters sometimes report a dreamlike and even paranoid experience that they would not otherwise routinely report.

A recent study (Liao et al., 2010) provided direct evidence of damage to white matter brain in the frontal and temporoparietal (front and side) areas among chronic adult users. The degree of damage is correlated with the severity of drug use.

49. How is cocaine used?

The medical uses of cocaine are now obsolete due to the development of more effective medications that have a lower or no potential for abuse. Cocaine is the most potent natural stimulant. It can be snorted, smoked, or injected. When combined with heroin and used by injection, it is called **speedballing**. The powder form is inhaled and thereby absorbed into the bloodstream through the nasal tissues. Injection into the veins introduces the drug directly with immediate euphoric effects. Inhaling the vapor through the lungs is as rapid as via injection. **Crack** is a cocaine base that comes in a rock crystal that is heated to produce vapors, which are smoked. The term *crack* refers to the crackling sound produced by the rock as it is heated.

50. What are LSD and PCP?

Lysergic acid diethylamide (LSD) and phencyclidine (PCP) are **hallucinogens**. Persons under the influence of hallucinogenic drugs often report seeing images, hearing sounds, and feeling sensations that seem real, but are not. Most of these substances are synthetically made to provide more potent effects. LSD is found in ergot, a fungus that grows on rye and other grains. PCP was initially used as an anesthetic but was discontinued because it caused agitation and delusions (false beliefs and paranoia) in patients. It can be snorted, smoked, or ingested. For smoking, PCP is often applied to a leafy material such as marijuana.

Other drugs in the hallucinogens class include psilocybin, mescaline, and foxy. Psilocybin is obtained from certain mushrooms found in South America, Mexico, and the United States. Once ingested, psilocybin is broken down to another hallucinogen, psilocin. Mescaline is the active hallucinogenic ingredient in peyote, a small, spineless cactus, which has been used for religious reasons by Mexican natives to induce mystical and spiritual experiences. Foxy, also known as foxy methoxy, is available in powder, capsule, and tablet form and is usually ingested orally.

Speedballing
Injecting a combination of cocaine and heroin.

Crack
A cocaine base that comes in a rock crystal that is heated to produce vapors, which are smoked. The term crack refers to the crackling sound produced by the rock as it is heated.

The term crack refers to the crackling sound produced by the rock as it is heated.

Hallucinogen
Drugs causing perceptual experiences that do not exist in actuality, including visual (seeing things) and auditory (hearing things) perceptions.

51. How is drug use related to other high-risk behaviors, like promiscuous sex?

Sexual development is an integral phase of adolescence that adolescents are expected to respond to in a healthy and responsible way. Drugs and sexual behavior can become intertwined. Drugs cause disinhibition that increases exposure to unsafe and nonconsensual sexual intercourse, leading to contraction of sexually transmitted diseases like gonorrhea, syphilis, chlamydia, hepatitis, and AIDS. It is also not unlikely that sexual intercourse can be a means for drug solicitation.

Among men, drug use is associated with earlier onset of sexual activity and increased lifetime sexual partners. A history of illicit drug use is related to decreased condom use (Galvez-Buccollini 2009), increasing the risk for sexually transmitted diseases.

PART SIX

Assessment and Diagnosis

How is drug abuse diagnosed?

Are any other tests involved in the drug abuse diagnosis process?

How long do drugs stay in the body? Is it true that marijuana stays in the body for about a month?

More . . .

52. How is drug abuse diagnosed?

Substance use and abuse falls on a continuum and the diagnosis of dependence and abuse can become arbitrary, especially in adolescents. In cases where symptoms do not meet the full criteria for the disorder, there is a risk to misinterpret those cases as less severe and thereby lose the opportunity for prevention efforts. This is more relevant in cases where risk factors are identified. The American Psychiatric Association's *Diagnostic and Statistical Manual (DSM) IV-TR* criteria are used to diagnose abuse and dependence among adolescents. Once dependence diagnosis is fulfilled for a specific drug, abuse diagnosis cannot be made, too.

Abuse, as defined by *DSM-IV* (APA, 1997) is a repetitive pattern of substance use resulting in significant impairment or distress to the individual, characterized by one (or more) of the following: failure to fulfill responsibilities at work, home, or school; usage of drug even when it is dangerous, such as before driving; continued drug use despite drug-related legal problems; and continued drug use despite negative consequences.

Substance dependence is characterized by a repetitive pattern of substance use resulting in significant impairment or distress to the individual. It has to fulfill at least three of the following criteria: tolerance (a reduced effect of the drug when used at the same amount or need for increased amounts of use to achieve the same high as a result of continued use); withdrawal (characteristic signs and symptoms manifest with cessation of drug use, or the same or similar drug is used to avoid or minimize withdrawal symptoms that occur as a result of repeated use); the use of more of the drug than that which is intended; the inability to control use of the drug; an increase in the amount of time spent obtaining the drugs or recovering from the effects of the drugs; the replacement of other activities with drug seeking behaviors; and continued use of the drug despite adverse consequences.

The presence of these criteria is necessary for at least one year for a diagnosis of substance abuse or dependence. If the criteria are met for less than a year, only a provisional diagnosis can be made. Criteria for substance dependence include several specifiers, one of which outlines whether substance dependence is with physiologic dependence (evidence of tolerance or withdrawal) or without physiologic dependence (no evidence of tolerance or withdrawal). In addition, remission categories are classified into four subtypes: (1) full, (2) early partial, (3) sustained, and (4) sustained partial, on the basis of whether any of the criteria for abuse or dependence has been met over a set time frame. The remission category also can be used for individuals receiving agonist therapy (such as methadone maintenance or suboxone) or for those living in a controlled, drug-free environment, including hospitals, inpatient drug rehabilitation programs, or therapeutic communities.

53. What do you mean by tolerance and withdrawal, especially for children?

Withdrawal from drugs, despite chronic use, is rare in adolescents, further supporting the cognitive distortion that a drug is not addictive.

Adolescents who have developed a tolerance for a drug will report to me that they have to use more often and usually at increasingly higher amounts to achieve the same high. Many adolescents, however, do not see this as evidence of dependence. In some cases, they will

Withdrawal from drugs, despite chronic use, is rare in adolescents, further supporting the cognitive distortion that a drug is not addictive.

eventually graduate to other drugs to achieve the same effects. Tolerance has some physiologic basis. The body, in particular, the receptors—molecular messengers in the brain—have been modified (such as an increase in numbers) such that the adolescent needs more drugs to occupy those receptors to achieve the same physiologic effects, or that secondary messengers that need to increase in amounts to achieve the same effects have developed.

Also, withdrawal has a physiologic basis in that brain receptors have been occupied long enough that removing drugs from them will cause a change in their configuration, thereby causing characteristic negative physical experiences. Presence of either tolerance or withdrawal, or both, define what is called a **physiologic dependence**. This is contrasted from loss of control (obsessive preoccupation) and the need to use without the necessary physiologic change. Known as psychological dependence, this dependence is manifested as craving or loss of sense of control over use. When this occurs, other drug-seeking behaviors are seen, like stealing money from family members, selling family possessions to buy drugs, drug dealing, and worse, prostitution.

Physiologic dependence

Changes in chemical messengers as evidenced by tolerance and withdrawal. Results from long-standing drug use.

54. Can you explain the 12-month period as part of a diagnosis?

Although a diagnosis of substance abuse or dependence is based on meeting the criteria for 12 months, adolescents can have significant problems even before reaching the 1-year cutoff. In cases where the full criteria are met except for the time criteria, a provisional diagnosis can be made.

55. Do drugs affect adolescents as they do adults?

What makes drug use in adolescents particularly troublesome is the rapid change and growth that an adolescent's brain is undergoing. Because of this, the brain of an adolescent is more sensitive to the effects of drug and alcohol use. As mentioned previously, peak prevalence of drug use is from ages 18 to 29 years, making the adolescent stage a critical period of vulnerability. Animal studies involving rats exposed to alcohol levels simulating adolescent alcohol consumption showed alterations in dopamine in the nucleus accumbens (see Question 60), as well as changes in sleep patterns even after only brief exposure to high alcohol levels.

The human brain has its own natural cannabinoid receptors. Based on a review of the available data, it is postulated that cannabis exposure during adolescence disrupts this system that affects the release of other chemical brain messengers, causing increased risk of disordered thinking, or psychosis.

Adolescents who use drugs regularly suffer impairments in psychosocial and academic functioning because they have very limited coping skills to fall back onto. The sequelae of drug use is what we see when they become adults as they continue to present with these problems.

56. How is a drug abuse or dependence diagnosis made?

The psychiatric interview remains the cornerstone of diagnosis and evaluation and has implications in treatment planning. The immediate goal is to determine whether the adolescent has used a single psychoactive substance or a combination, and whether abuse or dependence exists. A comprehensive evaluation also addresses the presence of coexisting psychiatric conditions and establishes whether psychiatric symptoms are direct results of psychoactive substances or exist in combination with other psychiatric disorders. This entails a robust knowledge of epidemiology, phenomenology (descriptions of illnesses), and course of psychiatric disorders.

To illustrate this by looking at ADHD and substance use disorder, a differentiation is based on establishing symptoms of inattention, hyperactivity, and impulsivity before onset of substance use. ADHD typically begins before the age of 7, and symptoms can be seen as early as kindergarten. In some cases, children are observed to be very hyper even during preschool, and I have encountered some who have been denied admission to day care. It is likewise important to establish a synthesized history from multiple sources. Information should be obtained about the student's functioning in school, relationships with peers and friends, and how he or she manages his or her leisure time.

Be patient and plan for these psychiatric evaluations to take a long time so that you can have a better hold on what is happening with your child.

57. Are any other tests involved in the drug abuse diagnosis process?

Use of structured and semistructured interviews helps further describe the extent and severity of substance use and its impact in multiple domains. Remember the

CRAFFT and CAGE questions (see Question 7)? There are also more extensive questionnaires that have been used both in physicians' offices and in research. For individuals who have complaints other than substance use, routine questions surrounding substance use and use of screening questionnaires avoid omitting an otherwise important coexisting condition. Once one is screened and drug abuse is found to be significant, a more thorough evaluation can be made. A drug use screening inventory screens multiple domains and identifies youth in need of further assessment. Self-reported and self-administered instruments are available in paper-and-pencil or computer-assisted versions. The Addiction Severity Index was used to create adolescent screens such as the Adolescent Problem Severity Index, the Adolescent Drug Abuse Diagnosis Instrument, and the Teen Addiction Severity Index. Other measures include the Adolescent Drug Abuse Diagnosis (ADAD), Adolescent Diagnostic Interview (ADI), Diagnostic Interview Schedule for Children (DISC), and Teen Addiction Severity Index (TASI). Self-administered tests include the Minnesota Multiphasic Personality Inventory-A (MMPI), Personal Experience Inventory (PEI), Personal Experience Inventory (PEI), Personal Experience Screening Questionnaire (PESQ), Problem Oriented Screening Instrument for Teenagers (POSIT), Drug Use Screening Inventory-Revised (DUSI-R), and Substance Abuse Subtle Screening Inventory (SASSI).

These questionnaires may not be routinely used by practitioners because they rely more on a clinical interview. These inventories increase reliability of subsequent psychiatric interviews. In addition, some of these scales can be readministered to determine improvements or positive response to treatment over time.

58. It is true that brain images (through CT scans and MRIs) can detect damage from drug use?

Although brain images can be used to detect brain conditions where there are structural changes, like masses or tumors, these tests are not used primarily to arrive at a psychiatric diagnosis. They are, however, extensively used to advance research in substance abuse. In fact, the use of functional imaging (seeing how the brain works in real time) among live volunteers has given us a better understanding of which parts of the brain are involved in addiction. The part of the brain that is strongly implicated in drug abuse involves the same circuitry (connections) that also underlies the things that make us feel good or drive us to feel better. These are the nucleus accumbens and ventral tegmental area.

59. Is drug abuse or dependence considered to be a brain disorder?

Yes, but saying this is in no way minimizing the contributions of family and social factors that interplay with the biology of addiction. Advances in the way we image the brain and even look at how the brain works among live research participants have opened up remarkable theories and postulates on how addiction works. The studies done through the National Institute of Mental Health established functional and chemical changes in the brain resulting from drug use.

60. What parts of the brain are affected?

There are a number of brain areas that are implicated in drug use. Two brain regions are most commonly associated with the reinforcing effects of drugs: the nucleus accumbens and the ventral tegmental area. Neurons made up of dopamine project from the ventral tegmental area to the nucleus accumbens, forming the central mesocorticolimbic dopamine system. They then project into the deeper areas of the brain (limbic system) to the amygdala and hippocampus. These areas are responsible for memory stores of emotionally laden stimuli. They also project into more superficial surfaces (the cortex) of the brain, which are responsible for how certain stimuli in the environment become more prominent. This explains the phenomenon of craving. Expectedly, these are also the same areas that are involved when we talk about the things that normally make us feel happy—when we get satisfied from food or eating chocolates, when being greeted by friends or families, or when watching our favorite programs on TV, listening to music, or having downtime with our families.

What changes for drug addicts is the way these usual sources of happiness become less reassuring, and drugs take a predominant role in these individuals. Addictive behavior is very much a part of the context of drug-seeking behavior. This is illustrated by cues in the environment that remind one of drugs to the extent of causing craving with psychological and bodily manifestations. Relapse has already started even before the resumption of use; that is, when individuals have experienced craving, they have relapsed.

Relapse has already started even before the resumption of use; that is, when individuals have experienced craving, they have relapsed.

Guia's comment:

I now know that addiction really causes brain changes. I grew up in a family where responsibility and choices were impor-tant. It is a matter of strong will and character, so if you are weak, you are more likely to use drugs. I realize now that it is not that simple. Having read and seen brain images with drug effects, I know that drugs affect the brain not only in how it functions but also in how the chemical messengers are altered. I am more realistic in dealing with my son's cravings.

61. Are there any brain messengers involved in drug use?

Yes. The most commonly implicated brain chemical mes-senger (neurotransmitter) is dopamine. This is the same chemical that lights up the brain when we eat chocolates, when we get praise, or feel happy being with friends. This is also involved with sexual satisfaction. Other chemical messengers and receptors (where the chemical messengers bind to exert their effects) include gamma hydroxybutyric acid, serotonin, nicotinic and choliner-gic receptors, and the N-methyl-D-aspartate systems.

62. How is drug testing done?

Monitoring of body fluids for the presence of substances is an important adjunct to treatment. Blood samples or gastric contents are tested during acute intoxication and in emergency room settings. Urine toxicology is more practical and is widely used to monitor response to treat-ment. Immunoassay techniques are useful screening tests, followed by gas chromatography/mass spectrometry for confirmation. Quantitative assay is useful to track reuse within a defined period of time.

Immunoassay is a biochemical test that involves measuring a property of the drug to be identified, called the analyte, to determine its presence or concentration. Assays are based on the ability of a substance to bind to the analyte, and an immunoassay can be qualitative or quantitative. A qualitative measurement consists of a sample without the analyte and one with the lowest concentration detectable, and a quantitative measurement requires references of known quantities.

Positive screening tests are then confirmed by gas chromatography/mass spectrometry. This procedure is considered the gold standard as it is a very specific test for the presence of a particular drug. They work synergistically to identify the substance compared to when either used separately. Gas chromatograph utilizes very fine columns through which different substances (drugs) pass through. Based on their intrinsic properties, these substances will travel along these tubes at varying elapsed times. The mass spectrometer will then capture these molecules and break them into charged (ionized) fragments which are then quantified.

Because "dirty" urines have far-reaching implications, sample collection is important. The following are suggested:

1. Removal of access to articles that promote adulteration (removal of articles of clothing used for concealment, water fountains, etc.)
2. Minimum of 60 milliliters (2 oz.) to prevent short sampling
3. Proper labeling and identification of sample
4. Proper documentation of the chain of custody

Random serial drug testing gives an objective measure of the individual's attempt at his or her sobriety. In addition, the testing serves as a deterrent to relapse. The aim is for the adolescent to eventually incorporate this sense of control as his or her own personal tool.

Hair sampling is not commonly used, but it is more sensitive and can detect drug use as far back as 3 months. Saliva and sweat can also be sampled.

63. I heard that kids could do something to make the sample read negative. Is this true? How is this detected?

You've probably heard that adolescents drink a lot of water to dilute the urine thinking that the drug test will then be negative. For the most part, what can more likely adulterate urine samples and render false positive results is what is *added* to it at the time of collection. Adulteration of urine samples generally fall into three categories: (1) urine substitution; (2) ingestion of fluids to dilute the sample or interfere with the testing process; and (3) direct adulteration of the sample itself. A pragmatic approach is to time urine sampling with random collections. A number of drugs are pH dependent, with excretion hastened when pH is lowered. Thus, consumption of cranberry or vinegar produces more of the drugs in the urine. Ingestion of large amounts of vitamins C, B, niacin, and goldenseal has been shown to be completely ineffective by various studies. Addition of sodium chloride, sodium bicarbonate, hydrogen peroxide, bleach, alcohol, blood, and soaps has been shown to produce false positive and false negative results. Obtaining samples can be stringent, and there are certain protocols that are followed to include one-on-one monitoring. Colorants may be placed in toilet bowls to make sure that samples are not adulterated by toilet water. Samples tested for legal purposes follow a chain of command that must be adhered to.

There are means to detect adulteration in the laboratory, including the following:

1. *Urine appearance and color*—Alcohol, soaps, and bleach are readily identified by odor. Soaps cause excessive bubbling. Solid adulterants are seen as residues in the container.

2. *Creatinine level*—The creatinine level is normally greater than 40 mg/dL; less than 20 mg/dL is abnormally diluted; this leads to false negative results.

3. *Specific gravity*—The level of specific gravity is normally between 1.002 and 1.030 g/ml. Extremely low specific gravity suggests dilution whereas a high specific gravity indicates dissolved solids.

4. *pH level*—The pH level is normally between 4.8 and 7.8. Low pH suggests acidic substances like cranberry juice and vinegar were ingested. Elevated pH suggests basic compounds like sodium bicarbonate and bleach were added to the urine.

5. *Detection of temperature*—Within 4 minutes of collection, the sample normally yields a temperature of 32.5 to 37.7°C. If it doesn't, it has probably been altered.

64. How long do drugs stay in the body? Is it true that marijuana stays in the body for about a month?

Cutoff levels for different drugs are established by individual laboratories to match analytical and client needs. For a test to be reported as positive, drugs must meet the **threshold concentration**, which is greater than the

Threshold concentration

The level of drug in a sample that meets or exceeds a preestablished cutoff level. A sample with a level above this concentration is said to be positive.

Limit of detection

The lowest level of drug at which an instrument is able to determine its presence.

Sensitivity

The proportion with which the presence of a drug is correctly identified in drug testing.

Limit of quantitation

The lowest level of drug at which its presence cannot be reliably determined.

limit of detection, also known as **sensitivity**, and usually greater than the **limit of quantitation**, the lowest level of accurate quantitation. Results are not reported as "negative," as this implies absence of drug being tested. Laboratories do not test down to a level of zero. "None detected" means that no drug is present or the drug is present but below the threshold concentration. Detection of drugs in the urine is dependent on a number of factors including variability of urine specimens, drug metabolism and half-life, patient's physical condition, fluid intake, and method and frequency of ingestion. **Table 2** provides time estimates with which drugs can be detected in the urine.

Marijuana can stay in your body for about a month if you are a regular user. A single use of marijuana may only persist for 4 days, such that urine testing after that time can have a negative result. It is customary to have urine

Table 2 Time Estimates of Drug Detection in Urine Samples

Drugs	Estimated Window of Detection (Days)
Amphetamines	1–3
Barbiturates (short/intermediate acting) Phenobarbital	2–4 Several weeks
Benzodiazepines	1–3
Cannabinoids	4–30
Cocaine	1–3
Ethanol	Less than 24 hours
Opiates (morphine and codeine)	2–3
Phencyclidine	2–3
Synthetic opioids	1–2

samples tested up to a maximum of 4 days of interval in between tests to reliably detect use. Adolescents often comment that they have only smoked marijuana once but that it will stay in their bodies for weeks. Marijuana gets stored in body fat, and prolonged storage is only through repeated use over longer periods of time. In addition, quantification gives a good time line of use and estimate of use in the last 30 days.

Rachelle's comments:

Kids would tell me that weed stays in the body for thirty days. Even for someone who had smoked a blunt only once, he or she will not stay positive for longer than a week. Persistence of the drug for at least thirty days with cessation of use indicates a pattern of regular use. The level of the drug that is present gives a good estimate of last use. This helps me to determine whether my son is forthcoming about his use or not.

65. What are the usual drugs for which one is tested?

The usual toxicology test includes tests for opioids, cocaine, and cannabis.

66. Can I use an over-the-counter screening kit?

Parents have reported using these kits and find them helpful. The kits will test for the following: marijuana, cocaine/crack, amphetamine (Ritalin, Dexedrine), meth-amphetamine (crystal meth), and morphine/opiates (heroin, codeine).

67. My son said he uses weed but he also tested positive for opioids and PCP. He insists he is not using them. Could he be telling the truth?

Occasionally, urine drug tests will be positive for both cannabis and opioids. During an interview, adolescents may repetitively deny that they are abusing heroin or opioids. This can also be attributed to cannabis laced with opioids, which is not their drug of choice. Sometimes, adolescents report heightened aggression or paranoia with cannabis intoxication. This can be attributed to cannabis laced with PCP. As PCP is not routinely tested, this is not regularly documented in reports unless there are strong reasons to also screen for it.

68. How will I know if the drug test results are accurate?

Once a specimen has been declared positive, it can be subjected to further confirmatory tests, which are at least 99% accurate.

Screenings depend on the cutoff for each particular drug tested, which is determined by federal standards. Once a specimen has been declared positive, it can be subjected to further confirmatory tests, which are at least 99% accurate. Thin-layer chromatography is highly specific for a particular drug being tested.

You may have heard adolescents who had tested positive say that they were with a group of kids who were using and that they did not smoke but inhaled the others' smoke second hand (close box). There is no evidence that this would result in a positive urine test. Studies have simulated a situation where individuals who did not smoke but were placed in a closed car with other individuals who smoked marijuana were tested, and they were found to have negative urine drug tests. I often hear this from adolescents as an excuse for positive test results while in treatment. It is simply not the case.

69. What are other drug tests?

Serum toxicology (blood samples) is also used, especially in emergency room settings. Other tests include breath-alyzer tests used by law enforcers, and less commonly used tests involving hair and saliva. The U.S. National Highway Traffic Safety Administration has considered breath alcohol devices approved for evidentiary use with results admissible in court. A word of caution: These tests are used in conjunction with other physical evidence like being able to walk on a straight line and good coordi-nation. I remember taking this test with my supervisor and a recent mouthwash gargle made my test positive!

70. What about alcohol strips? Can these be useful?

Parents of individuals in a day program (see Question 77) who use no drugs other than alcohol have found alco-hol strips helpful as a deterrent for relapse. As alcohol is not routinely tested, some individuals will even change their drug of choice from marijuana to alcohol to escape detection of drug use. Alcohol strips use saliva to detect presence of alcohol. Concentration of alcohol in saliva compared to blood is almost 1:1. A vendor has claimed sensitivity is up to 0.02% (http://www.ivdpretest.com/Alcohol-Saliva-Rapid-Test-Strips.html).

PART SEVEN

Treatment

What is the goal of treating my son?

How do I know how much treatment my child needs?

How can I be a part of my child's treatment?

What is Relapse Prevention?

More . . .

71. *Does drug treatment really work?*

It is encouraging that most interventions are effective. Large-scale studies demonstrated efficacy in terms of drug use reduction, criminality, and improved overall functioning. A very important aspect of treatment is the attitude of treating clinicians. Dealing with adolescents who have abused drugs creates special challenges and strong reactions even from treating providers, which can make treatment difficult at the outset. For the adolescent, this is particularly difficult, as engagement in treatment is significantly more erratic and dictated by outside forces.

A very important aspect of treatment is the attitude of treating clinicians.

The Cannabis Youth Treatment study evaluated the effectiveness and cost-effectiveness of five short-term outpatient interventions for adolescents who used cannabis. Treatment included Motivational Enhancement Therapy (see Question 90), Cognitive Behavioral Therapy (see Question 86), family education and therapy components (Family Support Network), an adolescent community reinforcement approach, and Multidimensional Family Therapy. Six hundred cannabis users also had other substance use, legal issues, and family issues. All five interventions demonstrated significant effects by decreasing drug use. The most cost-effective interventions were Motivational Enhancement Therapy, Cognitive Behavioral Therapy, and the adolescent community reinforcement approach (Dennis et al., 2004).

In 2009, another study large study demonstrated efficacy of treatment of substance abuse among adolescents with ADHD. This is very encouraging, as the study involved screening of 1334 youngsters, of whom 300 were included in the study. The study covered 11 sites across the country. To make the study as authentic as possible, it addressed the need to include as many individuals who are usually in community settings as possible in addition to those individuals who were only seen in hospital and study settings. As parents know, it is particularly challenging for adolescents to get engaged and be retained in treatment. Compliance of individuals in this study proved to be excellent—even better than those in the Cannabis Youth Treatment study. Because parents have expressed concern that stimulants can be abused, the Osmotic Release Oral System (OROS) methylphenidate (Concerta) was chosen to be used in this study because it is proven to have a good safety profile with a low abuse potential. Emergent side effects are usually mild and transient.

Melissa's comment:

I am more hopeful for my child. It's been difficult to even find help for my daughter. I don't know anything about drugs, or at least I didn't before we all got help. The professionals gave me options and, of course, I have done my own reading. There are treatments that specifically address the needs of my child and at the same time, help us to cope with her problems.

72. What is the goal of treating my son?

The goal is achieving and maintaining abstinence from drug use. Risk factors are identified, and areas of concern in psychopathology, social skills, family functioning, academic and school functioning, and involvement in prosocial activities stress the multidimensional approach to treatment. Treatment is therefore aimed at improving overall psychosocial functioning in addition to resolution of symptoms. It is important to assist him in fulfilling his developmental roles and expectations. As treatment can be on a longer term, his needs have to be met in the least restrictive level based on need.

73. What are the features of treatment facilities that I should look for?

Characteristics of treatment facilities should be intensive and sufficient enough to achieve changes in attitude and behavior; the duration of treatment depends on the severity of problems. There are ways to engage adolescents and retain them in treatment (see Motivational Enhancement Therapy in Question 90). Aftercare follow-up should be provided; this serves as a means to further help adolescents in applying learned skills once they are back in the real world. This also allows for extending the duration of treatment to support longer term sobriety. The program should be as comprehensive as possible and target psychosocial dysfunction in multiple areas. This includes treating coexisting psychiatric disorders; addressing vocational and educational needs; and providing recreational/leisure time activities, birth control services, and information about substance use/medical issues, particularly HIV/AIDS. In a number of situations, this may initially be the reason to hook youths into treatment. Facilities should also be sensitive to cultural issues; there are certain challenges that are particularly important to certain groups (Hispanics, Asian, African Americans, people from the Caribbean, those with issues of religion and spirituality, Anglo Saxons, etc.). They must encourage family involvement, which is a key component, especially with adolescents. I emphasize that parents need to be involved and know what is going on with their children's treatment, as not knowing what is happening can be used to undermine the treatment. Parents should form part of the individualized Relapse Prevention Plan that will be developed during treatment. Parents should feel at ease so that monitoring and checking their kids should come as naturally as possible. Lastly, facilities should have access to social services or case management, which can help the family link to additional services, especially during the aftercare planning.

74. Once an addict, always an addict. Is there any truth to this statement?

There is truth to this, which can be viewed as a double-edged sword. Some can view this in a negative way such that no recovery is possible. In order to be helpful in maintaining sobriety, one must believe recovery is possible. This is a reminder that individuals need to be vigilant and always on guard for any early relapse signs so that use or a full-blown relapse can be avoided. It is also important that following treatment, parents continue to be part of their child's sobriety through constant monitoring for any recurrence or early warning signs, which parents should have learned during their child's treatment.

75. Are there other things issues that should be addressed?

While medication has a role in treatment, it must be combined with counseling and skill building. This is particularly important as your child starts to hang out with his or her friends again, especially when it comes to learning to assert oneself. It is likely that he or she will have difficulty avoiding those who smoke weed or use drugs. Adolescents will need to be able to refuse drugs if offered, and even assert themselves to their friends and asking them to respect their sobriety by not using in their presence. Lack of problem solving, communication and interpersonal skills, and self esteem are, by themselves, identified as triggers for drug use that can be improved to lessen the likelihood of relapse. Ways to improve some of these skills are described in manuals or how-to books, though of course, improving these skills is facilitated by trained counselors. High-risk situations (situations that increase the likelihood of drug use) can be rehearsed in role plays so that ways to deal with these situations can be anticipated.

76. How do I know how much treatment my child needs?

Interventions need to be responsive to your child's needs. Levels of care depend on intensity of treatment services and supervision. These include inpatient treatment, residential treatment (group homes, therapeutic communities), partial hospitalization, or day treatment and outpatient treatment with or without community treatment (self-help groups or self-support groups). The American Society of Addiction Medicine has placement criteria for adolescents that take these variables into account during a comprehensive evaluation.

Duration of treatment is determined by likelihood of a successful transition to a lesser restrictive setting. Outpatient treatment is the least restrictive level whose treatment is time limited and focused. This usually involves a single or limited combination of treatment modalities.

Community treatment includes school-based programs and self-help groups such as Narcotics Anonymous (NA) or Alcoholics Anonymous (AA), which are important adjuncts to treatment. Self-help groups are available for families and friends (Al-Anon, Parents of Teenage Alcohol and Drug Abusers), which provide support, psychoeducation, and modeling to reduce maladaptive enabling behaviors of parents, families, and friends.

Lito's comment:

For my son, Stanley, being in a residential program stopped his drug use. He was using a lot of cough medications and got involved with legal problems. It was difficult for me to even consider that he had to go to a drug program. He was away from us and his siblings missed him. I believe now that he needed his own time alone to grow up and mature. He is now more confident and looks forward to going home, and I also feel more confident in helping him keep his sobriety.

77. What is a day program?

A **day program** is an outpatient program that is usually considered when your child's needs cannot be met by simply attending weekly individual or group counseling. A day program consists of providing milieu treatment (the setting becomes a driving force of treatment, with a built-in behavior plan), in addition to a number of group, family, and individual therapies. Certain programs also provide psychiatric treatment, with medication monitoring in particular. Day programs may either be after school or for a full day, depending on how intensive the needs are or how compromised the adolescent's functioning has been. For example, if the adolescent has been missing classes, has had multiple suspensions, or is failing in school, a full-day program is justified.

Day program

An intensive outpatient treatment program that relies heavily on milieu as its defining treatment, combined with behavior interventions, and group, individual, and family therapies.

Parental involvement is key to the success of this program. Parents have to make use of the behavior modification to effect positive changes in their child's behavior. This is an expectation that I always discuss with parents at the outset. Due to mounting frustration, parents

Parental involvement is key to the success of this program.

have the tendency to expect providers to treat their child without the parents being involved, and this is a limiting problem that has to be addressed.

78. When should I hospitalize my child?

The American Society of Addiction Medicine criteria have been modified to meet the needs of adolescents for placement purposes. Criteria for receiving inpatient treatment include:

1. Controlled environment for persistent running away
2. Separation from a problematic family environment so that crisis stabilization can be made in an inpatient setting
3. Increasing intensity of treatment when lower levels of care are not sufficient
4. Severe and clinically significant psychiatric conditions involving psychosis, suicidal or homicidal behavior, or acutely dangerous behavior
5. Risk of withdrawal problems

Adolescents with severe personality maladaptive patterns, inadequate psychosocial supports, and history of treatment failures are appropriate candidates for residential treatment.

79. How many adolescents have been treated in hospitals?

In 2006, there were 2.1 million youths aged 12–17 (8.2% of this population) who needed treatment for an illicit drug or alcohol use problem. From this, only 181,000 youths received treatment at a specialty facility (approximately 8.7% of youths who needed treatment), leaving 1.9 million youths who needed treatment for a substance use problem but did not receive it at a specialty facility. **Specialty treatment** is defined as treatment received at any of the following types of facilities: hospitals (inpatient only), drug/alcohol rehabilitation facilities (inpatient or outpatient), or mental health centers. It does not include treatment at an emergency room, private doctor's office, self-help group, prison, or jail.

In 2006, approximately 7.7% of the drug/alcohol admissions to treatment facilities in the United States involved individuals ages 17 and younger. Significantly, marijuana abuse ranks as the highest reason for admission at 61% of those admitted younger than 15 years and 65% of those admitted between 15 and 17 years. Alcohol abuse and alcohol abuse with secondary drug abuse is responsible for 7–12% of those admitted. Two to four percent of admission was accounted for by methamphetamine use.

Edwin's comments:

I realize that sometimes, hospitalization is necessary. My son Bobby was depressed and using drugs and I didn't know which one was driving the other. He was so depressed that he could not take care of himself, but he continued to use. The doctor recommended hospitalization to stabilize him, and I would have lost him without it. The hospital staff has been helpful. After that, he came back to the day program and continued to move on.

Specialty treatment

Treatment received at any of the following types of facilities: hospitals (inpatient only), drug/alcohol rehabilitation facilities (inpatient or outpatient), or mental health centers.

80. When should we consider residential programs for our daughter?

In cases where an adolescent needs long-term treatment, residential programs employing the principles of a therapeutic community (TC) can be considered. These are individuals with long-standing history of drug use, failed intensive programs, and those with legal problems. A number of adolescents are also court mandated to complete residential programs. There are also certain TC programs that incorporate psychiatric consultations to deal with treatment and diagnostic issues and also for medication evaluations. Some TCs are modified to meet the needs of special populations like mentally ill chemical abusers in community residences, adolescent substance abusers in residential TCs, and criminal offenders in corrections facilities.

The TC consists of staff with or without recovery experiences and provides a constellation of services including medical and mental health and vocational and educational services. Work and assigned job responsibilities are a means to therapy and improving interpersonal skills with both peers and authorities. Peers act as role models to expected behaviors. Staff members play the role of rational authority figures, providing feedback and direction. Those in the program are expected to work with the "program," which refers to following the structure and communication lines of the community and the "family" (clients and staff). The program follows a strict schedule of therapeutic, recreational, and educational activities. Encounters are the cornerstone of treatment. These are peer led, and participants are made aware of the behaviors that need to be modified. Probes, on the other hand, are staff led, with the goal of further understanding the individual's background for treatment planning purposes and also for fostering trust, openness, and support.

Some have even claimed that residential treatment does not work. To simply view residential treatment as a failure is to overlook a number of factors that have been identified that affect long-term outcomes, both positive and negative, and the corrective actions that have been incorporated by providers to directly address this gap. Because 60% of individuals relapse within 90 days of discharge from residential treatment, case management, coupled with assertive interventions, was designed to provide rapid initiation of continuing care in the community. This is part of the discharge planning that is done while still in treatment.

An important aspect of any treatment is to establish support that such interventions do in fact work when using clearly defined outcome measures. In the substance abuse field, there are a number of evidence-based interventions including Cognitive Behavior Therapy (CBT), Motivational Enhancement Therapy (MET), Community Reinforcement Approach (CRA, adapted for adolescents), and Contingency Management (CM). CRA is a comprehensive behavioral approach aimed at identifying factors in the environment that promote sobriety. It also involves skill building and developing prosocial skills that compete with drug-seeking behaviors. CM is differentially rewarding desired behaviors (sobriety) while punishing or withholding reinforcement for undesired behaviors (drug use). Positive reinforcers can include receiving vouchers or tokens if abstinence is exhibited and being placed on contract, bracelet monitoring, or house arrest for drug relapse. The challenge is for these proven treatments to be provided at varying levels of care from the traditional outpatient to day programming to levels as intensive as an inpatient setting or a residential program.

In a recent study (Garner et al., 2009), the Washington Circle (WC) continuity of care after long-term residential treatment performance measure was studied as well as the effect of assertive continuing care interventions in achieving continuity of care. The WC, which has been previously shown to be reliable with patients, was now tested to see if it can be generalized to a program level (residential treatment facility) whose treatment is reimbursed through public funding. Three hundred and forty-two adolescents who were admitted to long-term residential treatment were randomly assigned to either standard continuing care or an assertive continuing care condition (CRA, CM, or both). Because the study utilizes a randomized design, it experimentally tested the ability of the WC performance measure to predict outcome.

The following were measured: degree of substance-related problem, length of residential treatment, type of intervention, whether the intervention was with or without assertive conditions, presence or absence of follow-up within a two-week period after discharge from residential treatment, and recovery status (whether sober or not) while in the community.

Individuals included in the study were mostly adolescent Caucasians between 15 and 16 years old with significant legal involvement, high levels of dependence (mostly to cannabis and alcohol), and high co-occurring psychological problems and involvement in risky behaviors (multiple sexual partners and unprotected sex).

Those adolescents involved with WC have a significantly higher continuity of care treatment. Greater severity of the substance problem at baseline decreases the likelihood of recovery at three months. This emphasizes the need to provide ongoing effective substance abuse interventions by qualified and trained clinicians. Because there is a high degree of co-occurring psychological conditions, treatment also has to address these. Adolescents achieving continuity of care criteria had approximately a 92% chance of being sober at three-month follow-up compared with adolescents who did not achieve these criteria.

There are component treatments that do work. What is important is to provide these services concurrently in a coordinated manner from a multimodal and multidisciplinary approach and where case management is also provided. Meeting the needs of the adolescent should be guided by what can minimally meet his or her needs given a particular set of circumstances. Residential treatment may well be the least restrictive level meeting the youngster's needs at a particular time and this certainly needs to be periodically reviewed and revised accordingly as to whether criteria for this level of care are continually met.

81. I've heard about 12-steps programs. Are they for adults only?

Most Alcoholics Anonymous (AA) and Narcotics Anonymous (NA) groups are for adults, and adolescents may be unable to identify with what is going on in the meetings. Parents have even expressed concern that their sons and daughters will be influenced by hard-core drug addicts there. While these concerns can be valid, they illustrate that it is all the more important that parents help find the right fit for their children. The utility of these support groups can be more meaningful for adolescents who have already been introduced to them in prior treatments. Most of the interventions are provided in longer term treatments.

The 12-steps programs are rooted in the belief that recovery from addiction is only possible if one recognizes his problem with alcohol or drugs and admits that use of drugs in moderation is impossible without significant psychosocial consequences. The most widely used approach is based on the principle and philosophy of AA and NA. Treatment programs based on NA/AA models are also known as the Minnesota model or self-help programs. Adolescents are expected to finish the first three to five steps during inpatient or residential treatment. Concepts of acceptance, surrender, spirituality, and powerlessness may be difficult for adolescents to handle. The *Step Workbook for Adolescent Chemical Dependency Treatment* (Jaffe, 1990) offers a developmentally appropriate guide to the first five steps. Step 1 is the acknowledgment of inability to control substance use and is a confrontation of denial as well as developing motivation to participate in treatment. Steps 2 and 3 are also motivational in nature, emphasizing the need for help from someone other than the addict himself or herself. Adolescents are encouraged to look outside of themselves for guidance, structure, and meaning. Step 4 is the development of moral inventory involving a description of past behaviors. This lays the groundwork for subsequently dealing with issues identified. Step 5 explicitly asks for verbal disclosure and implicitly letting the adolescent deal with a helping individual. This modified approach still needs to be empirically tested.

Adolescents are encouraged to look outside of themselves for guidance, structure, and meaning.

82. Have the 12 steps been studied in adolescents?

Several studies on 12-step approaches were associated with positive treatment outcomes. Fiorentine (2000) found that adolescents with prior 12-step involvement remained in a substance abuse treatment program longer and were also more likely to complete treatment than those without such prior involvement. Both pretreatment 12-step meeting experience and longer duration of participation in drug treatment were positively associated with subsequent 12-step involvement. Adolescents who were involved in a combination of formal drug treatment and 12-step approaches were more likely to have high rates of abstinence than those who participated in either drug treatment or in a 12-step approach alone. Weekly or more frequent 12-step attendance was also associated with drug and alcohol abstinence (Fiorentine, 1999). A 12-step recovery support group combined with Relapse Prevention treatment resulted in an earlier decrease in drug use (Wells, Peterson, Gainey, Hawkins, & Catalano, 1994).

Adolescents who attended AA/NA meetings after substance abuse treatment have higher rates of abstinence and productivity compared with those who did not attend such meetings (Alford, Koehler, & Leonard, 1991). For adolescents who received inpatient substance abuse treatment, 12-step attendance was the most powerful predictor of drug abstinence at 6- and 12-month follow-up (Hsieh, Hoffmann, & Hollister, 1998).

In another study (Alford et al., 1991), adolescent inpatients who had a prior history of substance abuse treatment, more feelings of hopelessness, friends who did not use drugs, and less parental involvement while in treatment were more likely to attend AA than other adolescent inpatients. Three spirituality-related characteristics—feeling connected to others, frequency of meditation and prayer, and spiritual orientation to life—distinguished the subjects who expressed preference for both spirituality and 12-step approaches being integrated in TC treatment (Aromin et al., 2006).

83. How effective are group therapies?

Group therapy can be nonstructured or process-oriented groups aiming to break denial. Other goals include expressing and clarifying feelings, especially painful affective states, developing relationships, and confronting negative characteristics or behaviors impeding recovery. This is often confrontational. It seems that the adolescents with whom I work are more likely to believe other adolescents sharing similar experiences than the treating staff. A major hurdle for adolescents is the degree with which they will risk trusting others and disclosing personal information that they hold on to strongly.

84. How can I be a part of my child's treatment?

In previous questions, I have repeatedly touched on this. Family interventions are key components of adolescent substance abuse treatment as a number of family-related risk and protective factors have been identified. Commonalties in family treatment include psychoeducation about drug use, assisting families to initiate and maintain treatment of adolescents, and providing parent training to improve communication. Goals of family treatment include:

1. Decreasing the family's resistance to treatment
2. Redefining substance use as a family problem
3. Reestablishing parental influence
4. Interrupting dysfunctional sequences of family behavior
5. Assessing the interpersonal function of drug abuse
6. Implementing change strategies consistent with the family's interpersonal functioning
7. Providing assertive training skills for the adolescent and any high-risk sibling

It can be difficult to find programs that specifically provide these services. It is important to find those programs that can address these goals as described. A review of combined data on family literature showed its superiority over other modalities and also noted that it can enhance the effectiveness of other approaches. Treatment can involve all family members, as drug use is related to family dysfunctional relationships and interactional patterns. Examples of family treatment within this include multidimensional family therapy, multisystemic family therapy, and structural strategic family therapy. It is important to continue being a part of your child's treatment.

You need to empower yourselves to learn about drug use, how to monitor your children, know the early warning signs, and participate in scheduled family meetings and therapies. It may well be that you need to take a proactive role in pursuing family meetings with providers. To merely expect the provider to do the work and come back when your child has been "fixed" will not be beneficial to your child.

Jo's comments:

I realize that I have to be part of my child's treatment for it to work. I got angry after finding out that my son John was using. I gave him everything, and being a single mother, it has been tough for me to provide the things he needs and wants. I feel betrayed. When I decided to bring him for treatment, my attitude was like "Fix him. I've been there for him; this time, he needs to do this on his own." I now realize that as the parent, I also undergo adjustment. If anything, he now needs me more than ever. I have to heal with him.

85. What is multisystemic family therapy?

Multisystemic family therapy takes into account broader social relationships including teachers, neighbors, and other social units interacting with the drug-dependent adolescent. It is often incorporated in outpatient community-based settings and also includes case management. Treatment is made accessible to the families and is provided where they live. Case managers work with the families and other involved individuals like probation and parole officers and school officials. Adolescents are also provided with vocational services. The goal is to keep the adolescent in the community in which he lives and keep him in school. This family intervention has been most successfully applied among juvenile legal offenders and has not been routinely applied in traditional outpatient settings.

86. What is Cognitive Behavior Therapy?

Cognitive Behavior Therapy uses cognitive and behavioral interventions in changing faulty cognitions, which

Multisystemic family therapy

Treatment that takes into account broader social relationships including teachers, neighbors, and other social units interacting with the drug-dependent adolescent. The goal is to keep the adolescent in the community in which he lives and keep him in school. This is a very intensive treatment that has been supported to meet the needs of youngsters with multiple issues and legal problems.

Cognitive Behavior Therapy

Therapy that uses cognitive and behavioral interventions to improve skills and change maladaptive behaviors, which hinder cessation of drug use.

hinder cessation of drug use and improving skills. Social skills training addresses the following:

1. Consequential thinking to identify the antecedents and consequences of substance use behavior
2. Self-control in resisting impulse to use substances and peer pressure and to develop drug refusal skills
3. Avoiding trouble by identifying and avoiding high-risk situations for substance use and associated problem behaviors
4. Social networking by identifying prosocial activities and new, nonsubstance-using friends
5. Coping with authority by using negotiation and compliance skills
6. Problem solving for effective and prosocial solutions in difficult situations
7. Relapse coping by developing strategies for dealing with subsequent substance use behavior

87. What is Relapse Prevention?

Relapse Prevention is a cognitive behavioral approach aimed at developing self-control; identifying triggers in the environment leading to use and relapse; and developing coping skills in dealing with stressors, triggers, and lapses into substance use.

The individualized Relapse Prevention plan incorporates family responsibilties in supporting the child's sobriety.

88. What is a harm-reduction approach?

Harm reduction is a comprehensive philosophy used to decrease the negative effects of drug use on society. It

Relapse Prevention

A cognitive behavioral treatment approach aimed at developing self-control; identifying triggers in the environment leading to use and relapse; and developing coping skills in dealing with stressors, triggers, and lapses into substance use.

Harm-reduction approach

Treatment approach that consists of strategies in minimizing the impact of alcohol use and other high-risk behaviors. It operates on the theory that abstinence and minimal harm are goals, but proponents also recognize that any behavior changes that reduce harm are, by themselves, positive outcomes.

presupposes that a society has to deal with the presence of drug use because it can never be totally eradicated. Some may even see harm reduction as the end of or a means to abstinence and by no means should be viewed as a tool of drug legalization.

Principles of harm reduction have been applied in situations that have generated responses ranging from endorsement to protest and controversy. Harm reduction approaches include the Methadone Maintenance Treatment Program's aim at decreasing opioid use, delinquency, criminality and health problems; exchange needle programs to decrease HIV transmission; decriminalization of cannabis use in certain states and countries like the Netherlands to address illicit use and its legal consequences; and education and outreach on opioid overdose preventions.

89. Does harm reduction make drug use acceptable?

Motivational Enhancement Therapy

A type of evidence-based, non-coercive, and self-centered psychotherapy aimed at increasing the likelihood to change behaviors. As it applies to addiction, Motivational Enhancement Therapy increases the imbalance toward accepting the need to change from drug-seeking to non-using behaviors.

It would seem so, but only temporarily. Harm reduction can be seen as a means to the goal of full abstinence. If adolescents can achieve one goal at a time, starting with a decrease in drug use, then a decrease rather than cessation itself will be a step to the goal. This approach will allow adolescents to set realistic goals that they are able to achieve with concrete results.

90. What is Motivational Enhancement Therapy?

In Question 73, I mentioned **Motivational Enhancement Therapy** (MET) as a means to further engage adolescents in treatment and retain them. MET is a systematic intervention approach, based on the principles of motivational psychology, that is designed to produce rapid change whose underlying motivation comes from within the individual. Rather than being therapist driven, motivational strategies are used to facilitate an individual's own change. Motivational Enhancement Therapy arose from practical issues raised by clinicians in dealing with substance use, especially with people who are reluctant or ambivalent to change. Strategies are persuasive rather than coercive. It creates dissonance that is conducive to change. The overall goal is to increase intrinsic motivation. Five general principles are:

1. Express empathy as the adolescents do not see any problem with using

2. Develop discrepancy; present the pros and cons of drug use and tilt the arguments against use

3. Avoid argumentation—avoid direct confrontation and challenges

4. Roll with resistance, accepting the current level of resistance to treatment and lack of motivation thereof

5. Support self-efficacy; the adolescent will have the final say to make the change

91. I am opposed to medications. When should I consider medication for my child?

Very frequently, parents express opposition to medication in general. There is limited success in the use of medication to effect abstinence. This is especially the case when dealing with adolescents. In addition, most studies are based on adults. Even fewer case studies mentioned the use of medications to decrease craving.

Medications are clearly helpful in treating symptoms of withdrawal from certain drugs like alcohol, opioids, and benzodiazepines, and use of methadone or buprenorphine (Suboxone) is helpful as a detoxification medication or for maintenance. Medications can also be very helpful if drug use is also comorbid with moderate to severe depression, anxiety, psychosis, and ADHD. In fact, to resist aggressively treating these comorbid conditions can result in continued drug use. These conditions have to be treated aggressively and concurrently, and the adolescent will likely need a combination of treatments (medications and psychotherapy) on a long term. Physicians make use of medications for the following reasons:

1. To treat comorbid psychiatric disorders (stimulants for ADHD)
2. To take advantage of drug-aversive agents (like disulfiram for alcoholism)
3. To treat withdrawal effects (methadone for heroin or opioids)
4. To block reinforcing effect of drugs (buprenorphine for opioids)
5. To substitute a similar drug for prolonged maintenance (methadone for opioids)
6. To treat craving (modafinil for cocaine)

Substitution therapies and aversive agents are infrequently used in adolescents. However, if these medications can increase the likelihood of treatment success or at least prevent further problems, parents should discuss these options with the physician. Parents are hesitant about considering medications to treat substance abuse without coexisting psychiatric conditions in their children. While studies are limited, use of medications to treat substance abuse without coexisting psychiatric conditions is *safe* and *effective*. Nicotine patches have worked and have few side effects. Bupropion (Wellbutrin) has been used for adolescent nicotine addiction, ADHD, and depression. Buprenorphine (with or without naltrexone [Subutex or Suboxone]) has been studied and found to be safe and effective for adolescents who abuse opioids. Other medications that have been used and studied include medications that decrease craving for alcohol like disulfiram (Antabuse), naltrexone (Revia), acamprosate (Campral), and topiramate (Topamax), a medication used for seizures and bipolar disorder.

There are experimental drugs that are currently being investigated, including rimonabant and ondansetron for marijuana abuse.

Edith's comments:
I see that my son really needs his bipolar medication. John goes through ups and downs and he would smoke weed to bring himself down. He also experimented with cocaine. With Lithium, his mood became stable and he stopped using. Hopefully, it will be longer this time.

92. Are stimulants considered drugs?

Parents have commented that using stimulants to treat ADHD with drugs is using one addictive medication to treat another addiction. On the contrary, studies have shown that the use of stimulants to treat ADHD decreases risk of subsequent drug abuse or if abuse has already occurred, that it decreases relapse. There are anecdotal reports of kids misusing and abusing their stimulant medications. In my practice, I consider using nonstimulant medications to treat ADHD comorbid with drug use to address these concerns. This includes

Parents have commented that using stimulants to treat ADHD with drugs is using one addictive medication to treat another addiction.

atomoxetine (Strattera, a nonstimulant medication approved for ADHD) and bupropion (Wellbutrin, an antidepressant medication with some evidence of efficacy for ADHD). If stimulants have to be tried for lack of response to these medications, I consider Concerta (methylphenidate). Its preparation (in capsule OROS form) makes it difficult to pulverize and snort it.

There is a new medication called lisdexamfetamine, a prostimulant, that is converted to its active form, d-amphetamine, in the gut, and it has low abuse potential if taken intranasally or intravenously.

Diversion

Occurs when prescribed medications with addictive potential are made available to individuals for the sole purpose of getting high.

Stimulant misuse and **diversion** occurs in about 10–20% of college students surveyed. Stimulants are usually diverted from friends and used primarily to improve concentration and alertness in class rather than to get high.

93. I have heard that Subutex (buprenorphine) is used to treat heroin addiction. Does this method work?

Yes, and an additional benefit is that physicians with the proper training and authorization are now allowed to treat individuals with opioid addiction in an office setting. These individuals are usually able to keep their jobs and stay in school and can be seen monthly on a regular basis. I have treated youngsters with this medication. Buprenorphine, a partial agonist, can be used for **detoxification** (treatment of withdrawal symptoms), as an anticraving agent, and as a maintenance medication (to prevent relapse). Buprenorphine is also combined with naloxone (Suboxone) to decrease abuse and diversion. These medications are administered by placing them under the tongue. Being on buprenorphine is similar

Detoxification

Treatment of drug withdrawal symptoms, of which the level of medical supervision varies with the presence of life-threatening conditions or coexisting medical conditions.

to being on methadone (methadone maintenance treatment program), which also prevents relapse to drug use.

94. How is buprenorphine treatment different from methadone maintenance treatment programs?

Table 3 summarizes the features of the two types of outpatient opioid treatment.

95. Is disulfiram (Antabuse) safe to use in adolescents?

Disulfiram has been used in adolescents and was found to be safe and effective. When someone takes disulfiram and then consumes alcohol, he or she experiences uncomfortable body reactions, thus encouraging one to abstain from the consumption of alcohol to avoid these effects. Disulfiram produces symptoms of headache, flushing, nausea or vomiting, diarrhea, and blood pressure changes after consuming alcohol. There has been one good study that established that disulfiram has few side effects and those who received active treatment had longer duration of sobriety. It is usually given at 250 mg daily orally. Disulfiram should not be taken by those with liver problems.

96. How long will my child stay on medication? How long should my child be in treatment?

This is based on a number of factors, including need for maintenance medication (for example, recurrent depression or chronic psychosis) and presence of a stable support

Table 3 Community-Based Opioid Treatments

Features	Office-Based Buprenorphine Opiate Treatment (OBOT)	Methadone Maintenance Treatment Program (MMTP) Clinic
Medication	Buprenorphine (Subutex), a partial agonist, and Buprenorphine and Naloxone (Suboxone), a full antagonist, are placed under the tongue (sublingually). Naloxone is a medication with no reinforcing effects that is combined with Buprenorphine to avoid diversion and attenuate the reinforcing effects of Buprenorphine if abused, especially when injected.	Methadone is a synthetic full opioid agonist in liquid form that is taken orally. Patients take the medication as administered by a nursing staff through direct observation. This is in *contrast* to clinics that provide methadone for pain management. Dosing is determined by the prescribing MD—when patients get admitted to a hospital, verification with the MMTP Clinic is necessary to receive the prescribed dose; otherwise a maximum dose of 20 mg daily is given pre-verification to avoid a potential overdose. A lesser preferred medication, Levo-Alpha Acetyl Methadol (LAAM), is longer acting and can be given three times a week.
Schedule	III	II
Dosing	Induction is started at 2 mg and is increased every hour up to a maximum of 8 mg on day 1. Maintenance dose is achieved with cessation of withdrawal symptoms. Recommended dose can be up to 32 mg/day, mostly attained at 16–32 mg/day.	Titrated up to the dose covering withdrawal symptoms; can be increased if with craving. Usual dose is 60–80 mg daily.
Supply	Can be prescribed and dispensed by a physician. Can be given one week at a time during titration, and increased to a monthly supply.	Daily observed dosing. Some programs provide a weekend supply for established patients with good compliance and sobriety as well as safe methadone handling.
Uses	Opioid detoxification, initially used for induction. Dose is increased to cover withdrawal symptoms. Medication is then slowly tapered until discontinuation. Maintenance medication: Dose that covered withdrawal symptoms is continued for some time as the individual attains more stability in other areas (interpersonal, economic, educational, occupational). Individuals can then opt to be tapered until discontinuation. Also used to address craving.	Opioid detoxification, done in a medically supervised setting is initially used for induction. Dose is increased to cover withdrawal symptoms, then medication is slowly tapered until discontinuation. Maintenance medication: This is initiated only in MMTP clinics following a referral. Individuals are usually maintained for a longer period, such as years. Also used to address craving.

Setting	Office-based physician practice; periodic visits with drug testing and medication management; a maximum of 100 patients per physician. If treatment cannot support a patient's sobriety, the physician has to have ready access to referral (usually to an MMTP Clinic).	Dispensing medication is part of the responsibility of a comprehensive substance abuse clinic staffed by a physician, nurse, pharmacist, therapists, and substance abuse counselor. In addition to medication, counseling services include individual psychotherapy, group therapy, family therapy, and ancillary services like vocational training and psychiatric/medical services. Intensity of service decreases with increasing stability. Stable patients can be referred to OBOT clinics as appropriate (for example, patient shows no evidence of active substance abuse, is gainfully employed, and has psychiatric stability).
Requirements	Physician minimally needs an active medical license and DEA number. In addition, physician has to finish an 8-hour training and receive a waiver, and needs a special buprenorphine DEA number.	At minimum, physician needs an active medical license and DEA number.
Regulation	Under DEA oversight. Documentation of dispensing and administration of medications.	Stricter federal guidelines and regulations. Staffing is defined by regulations.
Advantages	Least disruptive to individuals needing treatment and still able to maintain employment; more suitable to adolescents who attend school.	Addresses patients who have multiple needs (medical, psychosocial, psychiatric).

Full Agonist: A chemical that binds to a receptor and exerts its full effect
Partial Agonist: A chemical that binds to a receptor and exerts less than its full effect
Antagonist: A chemical that binds to a receptor reversing the activity or exerting the opposite effect

system to effect longer-term sobriety, transition to school, or going back to school after a longer term treatment. For those who have coexisting psychiatric conditions, it is best to continue on maintenance medications.

In cases of depression, the following conditions favor use of medications for more than a year: recurrent depression (two depressive episodes or more), double depression (those with dysthymia and major depression, as reported by youngsters that they have been depressed "for as long as I can remember"), disordered thinking (psychosis), suicidal behavior, and ongoing family dysfunction. The goal of treatment is to gain full remission of symptoms and functioning and is no longer improvement of symptoms alone.

Parents should keep in mind that drug dependence is a chronic condition, so their child's use of maintenance medications is akin to those one might take for diabetes, asthma, or psychiatric conditions like recurrent depression, ADHD, and bipolar disorder. Part of medication monitoring is looking for long-term side effects of prescribed medications. Of note, some medications used to maintain remission of psychosis and bipolar disorder can cause weight gain, difficulties in managing sugar in the body, or increase in fats. Parents, families, and treating physicians should continue to discuss the need for these medications. I always encourage people to look for answers and questions so that active discussion and collaboration will continue.

97. What are the common side effects of medications?

The side effects are based on classes of medications such as those used for depression, psychosis, anxiety, and ADHD. **Table 4** gives an overview of general classes of medications, conditions for which they are prescribed, and common side effects.

The FDA has approved some medications for certain conditions in adults, and child psychiatrists use these medications to treat similar conditions in adolescents. These medications have few side effects and are effective. These are acceptable practices known as **off labeling**.

Off labeling

Use of medications under one of the following conditions: 1) prescription of an FDA-approved medication outside of its recommended dosage (a physician prescribes higher doses that what is recommended for an approved antidepressant), 2) prescription to an individual in a group for whom the drug was not studied (an approved antidepressant for adults being prescribed to adolescents), or 3) prescription of an approved medication for something other than what is was originally intended for (use of antidepressants for anger control instead of depression). This is an acceptable medical practice that requires full disclosure from physicians to parents to ensure that informed consent is obtained.

Table 4 General Overview of Classes of Medications Used to Treat Common Psychological Conditions

Classes	Indication	Common Side Effects
Selective Serotonin Reuptake Inhibitor (SSRI) (like fluoxetine, sertraline, citalopram)	Depression, Anxiety	Stomach upset, restlessness
Selective Norepinephrine Reuptake Inhibitor (SNRI) (like venlafaxine, duloxetine)	Depression, Anxiety	Stomach upset, restlessness
Atypicals (like Risperidone, Quetiapine, Olanzapine)	Psychosis, Bipolar Disorder	Drowsiness; extrapyramidal side effects such as stiffness, drooling, slowing sudden involuntary movements (acute dystonias), weight gain, impaired sugar metabolism (metabolic syndrome)
Stimulants: methylphenidate (Ritalin, Focalin, Concerta), Vyvanse, Methamphetamines (Adderall, Desoxygradumet)	ADHD	Restlessness, cardiac problems, tics
Nonstimulants: Atomoxetine (Strattera) Buproprion (Wellbutrin) Modafanil (Provigil)	ADHD	Drowsiness, anxiety

Premedication evaluations and workups are done to make sure that these medications are safe. Also, your child's physician will closely monitor your child. Your child's psychiatrist, who is preferably a child and adolescent psychiatrist with training in addiction, is best suited to answer your questions and concerns.

In order to ensure that medications are safe, the following are usually requested before trying a medication: a physical examination (usually done by the child's own physician) to identify any problems, and a laboratory examination involving the kidneys, blood, and liver, and in cases where stimulants are being considered, heart tracing or electrocardiogram. Studies have shown that stimulant use is correlated with (but not established as causing) sudden cardiac death in children and adolescents. The risk is increased if your child has structural heart abnormalities (enlarged or small heart, holes, or irregular heartbeat). Your child's physician will ask you if any risk factors are present, such as family history of heart disease, rhythm abnormalities (irregular heartbeat), or sudden death from heart attacks.

98. Is my son at risk for suicide while taking antidepressants?

The FDA has mandated drug manufacturers to issue a black box warning on antidepressants to monitor for suicidal behavior. A black box warning appears on the prescription label of a medication, indicating the significant, serious, or even potentially life threatening side effect(s) of that medication. This is the most serious warning required by the FDA, and it has also been applied to medications other than antidepressants. Certain antibiotics, such as ciprofloxacin, had a black box warning for swelling of tendons and rupture as a side effect resulting in permanent disability; and the diabetes medication rosiglitazone can cause significant heart problems. The black box warning for antidepressants has created considerable concern for parents, who do not want to give their child a medication that will worsen his or her depression. This warning was initially considered for antidepressants in 2004 after the FDA reviewed 23 studies involving more than 4300 children who received nine types of antidepressants and reported general characteristics of suicidal thinking and behavior. In 17 out of the 23 studies, asking about suicidal thoughts and behaviors was specifically included. In these data, medication did not worsen preexisting suicidal thoughts nor result in emergence of suicidal thoughts after treatment, and none of these individuals committed suicide (Parents Medguide for Depression). American studies have been done to further investigate this issue. One study (Simon, Savarino, Operskalski, & Wang, 2006) found that the risk for suicide was highest before medication treatment and significantly declined thereafter. Another study (Gibbons , Hur, Bhaumik, & Mann, 2006) found an association between higher SSRI prescription rates and lower suicide rates in children and adolescents.

Before the warning was given, there was an increasing trend in pediatric diagnosis of depression from 1993 to 2004. After that, there was a decrease in the diagnosis of depression, which deviated from what could have been predicted from the trend established in previous years. Pediatricians and nonpediatrician primary care doctors accounted for a reduction of these diagnoses. In 2002, 260 deaths from suicide occurred between the ages of 10 to 14 years, ranked third after accidents and malignancy as the leading cause of death in this age group.

From 1990 to 2003, the combined suicide rate among those aged 10 to 24 years declined 28.5%. However, from 2003 to 2004, the rate increased by 8.0%, the largest increase in a single year from 1990 to 2004 (CDC, 2007). Some believe this observation was correlated with a decrease in antidepressant prescription during that period. Treatment of pediatric depression with antidepressants declined significantly two years after this warning was given without any concomitant increase in the use of other treatments like counseling or use of other medication (Libby et al., 2007). In another follow-up study published two years later (Libby, Orton, & Valuck,

2009), underdiagnosis of depression persisted for both pediatric and adult patients, suggesting that the effects were persistent, significant, and covered not only minors but adult patients as well.

It is important to be informed about these issues; to be involved with your child's treatment; and to discuss these concerns with his or her psychiatrist, preferably a child and adolescent psychiatrist, who is best able to address these questions with you.

99. My son refuses to go into treatment. What should I do?

Adolescents who refuse treatment usually do not see their drug use as a problem and see no need to stop. Also, they may still have yet to see the negative consequences of drug use. There are certain interventions that deal with improving the motivation to change, called Motivational Enhancement Therapy. In certain cases, external leverage may need to come from concerned agencies to make them receive treatment. Some parents may even see these as counterproductive. The idea of getting adolescents into treatment is to work on improving their motivation. Engagement in treatment also allows disrupting the cycle of continued use. Adolescents will often continue to deny problems resulting from drug use. In these cases, it can be necessary to ask for additional external leverage by referring them to agencies like the Youth Services Bureau (YSB). The YSB is a government social services agency that provides prevention programs and treatment to families and youth at risk for delinquent behavior. The YSB may compel the youngster to get into treatment to avoid having to go to court or being placed in detention.

Recalcitrant and persistent drug use is an indication for inpatient admission. As parents, you may sign in your minor for treatment. This is where the family can rally together. That family member whom the youngster has identified to be most supportive of him or her can reinforce this decision. I have seen time and again adolescents who were admitted after vehemently refusing treatment say that this experience has helped them. Admission disrupted the cycle of use. It also allowed for providing necessary family interventions and increasing readiness for continuing aftercare treatment.

100. I have used drugs before and I'm using them again; I'm at a loss about what to do. Where can I get help?

This is one of the sensitive things that will have to be dealt with at some point during counseling. Parents will inevitably blame themselves once they find out that their children have used drugs. It is best to deal with family issues in a straightforward and honest way, and at the same time, also work with your child in dealing with his treatment. Partnership for a Drug-Free America has very good tips on how to talk to your kids about this.

It is important for parents to receive concurrent help to deal with their own sobriety. For parents who do not live with their substance-abusing adolescent, it is a bigger challenge to get them help. In this case, responsibility falls heavily on working with the adolescent in strengthening his or her self efficacy. It is doubly difficult to expect kids to stop using when their parents are not sober.

Eleanor's comments:

Having information about drugs has been helpful. Kush, haze, E, L, purple haze—words that come straight from kids. The Web sites are helpful in separating facts from myths.

Conclusion

Resources for parents who have children abusing drugs or for those who suspect as much include *Suspect Your Teen Is Using Drugs or Drinking? A Brief Guide to Action for Parents* (available at: http://ncadistore.samhsa.gov/catalog/ProductDetails.aspx?ProductID=16746), the Partnership for a Drug-Free America's *Helping Others With a Drug Problem* (available at: http://www.drugfree.org/Intervention/HelpingOthers), and the Substance Abuse and Mental Health Services Administration's *A Family Guide to Keeping Youth Mentally Healthy and Drug-Free* Web site (available at: http://family.samhsa.gov). The Substance Abuse and Mental Health Services Administration also has a telephone hotline and Web site to assist in identifying drug treatment programs throughout the United States. The number is 1-800-662-HELP. The treatment facility locator is available at http://dasis3.samhsa.gov. See the resources list in this book for contact information on these and other resources.

By reading this book, you should have recognized that drug abuse should be treated as a disorder with onset during adolescence, and it needs to be treated aggressively and early. Remember, drug use causes lasting negative effects with serious psychosocial and legal consequences for your developing child. Receiving treatment now will make a difference in your child's life and yours, *and it can be done!*

Appendix A: Resources

American Academy of Addiction Psychiatry (AAAP)
400 Massasoit Avenue
Suite 307, 2nd Floor
East Providence, RI 02914
Phone: 401-524-3076
Fax: 401-272-0922
www.aaap.org

American Academy of Child and Adolescent Psychiatry (AACAP)
P.O. Box 96106
Washington, DC 20016
Phone: 202-966-7300
Fax: 202-966-2891
www.aacap.org

American Society of Addiction Medicine (ASAM)
4601 N. Park Avenue, Upper Arcade No. 101
Chevy Chase, MD 20815
Phone: 301-656-3920
Fax: 301-656-3815
E-mail: email@asam.org
www.asam.org

Cocaine Anonymous World Services
21720 S. Wilmington Avenue, Suite 304
Long Beach, CA 90810-1641
Phone: 310-559-5833
Fax: 310-559-2554
E-mail: cawso@ca.org
www.ca.org

Drug Enforcement Administration (DEA)
www.justice.gov/dea/contactinfo.htm

**National Institute on Alcohol Abuse and Alcoholism
(NIAAA)**
5635 Fishers Lane, MSC 9304
Bethesda, MD 20892-9304
www.niaaa.nih.gov

National Institute on Drug Abuse (NIDA)
6001 Executive Boulevard, Room 5213
Bethesda, MD 20892-9561
Phone: 301-443-1124 (240-221-4007 en español)
E-mail: information@nida.nih.gov
www.nida.nih.gov

Office of National Drug Control Policy
Drug Policy Information Clearinghouse
P.O. Box 6000
Rockville, MD 20849-6000
Phone: 800-666-3332
Fax: 301-519-5212
www.whitehousedrugpolicy.gov

Partnership for a Drug-Free America
352 Park Avenue South, 9th Floor
New York, NY 10010
Phone: 212-922-1560
Fax: 212-922-1570
www.drugfree.org

**Substance Abuse and Mental Health Services
   Administration (SAMHSA)**
SAMHSA's Health Information Network
P.O. Box 2345
Rockville, MD 20847-2345
Phone: 877-726-4727
24-hour help line: 800-662-4357
Fax: 240-221-4292
E-mail: SAMHSAInfo@samhsa.hhs.gov
www.samhsa.gov

US Screening Source, Inc.
P.O. Box 22674
Louisville, KY 40252-0674
Phone: 866-323-7336
www.usscreeningsource.com/druginformation.htm

Appendix B:
Further Reading

Alford, G. S., Koehler, R. A., & Leonard, J. (1991). Alcoholics Anonymous-Narcotics Anonymous model inpatient treatment of chemically dependent adolescents: A 2-year outcome study. *Journal of Studies on Alcohol, 52,* 118–126.

American Psychiatric Association. (1994). *Diagnostic and Statistical Manual of Mental Disorders* (4th Ed.). Washington, DC.

American Psychiatric Association, American Academy of Child and Adolescent Psychiatry, & A National Coalition of Concerned Parents, Providers, and Professional Associations. The use of medication in treating childhood and adolescent depression: Information for patients and families. Retrieved from http://www.psych.org/Share/Parents-Med-Guide/Medication-Guides/ParentsMedGuide-Depression-English.aspx

Amethyst Initiative. Retrieved from www.amethystinitiative.org

Anderson, J. C., Williams, S., McGee, R., & Silva, P. A. (1987). DSM III disorders in pre-adolescent children: Prevalence in large sample from the general population. *Archives of General Psychiatry, 44,* 69–76.

Angold, A., & Costello, E. J. (1993). Depressive comorbidity in children and adolescents: Empirical, theoretical and methodological issues. *American Journal of Psychiatry, 150,* 1779–1791.

Anthony, J., & Helzer J. (1991). Syndromes of drug abuse and dependence. In L. Robins & D. Reiger (Eds.), *Psychiatric disorders in America* (pp. 116–154). New York, NY: Free Press.

Aromin, R. A., Galanter, M., Solhkhah, R., Bunt, G., & Dermatis, H. (2006). Preference for spirituality and twelve-step-oriented approaches among adolescents in a residential therapeutic community. *Journal of Addictive Diseases, 25*(2), 89–96.

Baer, J. S., MacLean, M. G., & Marlatt, G. A. (1998). Linking etiology and treatment for adolescent substance abuse: Toward a better match. In R. Jessor (Ed.), *New perspectives on adolescent risk behavior* (pp. 182–220). New York, NY: Cambridge University Press.

Blackson, T. C. (1994). Temperament: A salient correlate of risk factors for alcohol and drug abuse. *Drug and Alcohol Dependence, 36,* 205–214.

Bossong, M. G., & Niesink, R. J. (2010). Adolescent brain maturation, the endogenous cannabinoid system and the neurobiology of cannabis-induced schizophrenia. *Progress in Neurobiology*, 2010 Jul 15. (Epub ahead of print).

Brown, S. A. (1993). Recovery patterns in adolescent substance abuse. In J. S. Baer, G. A. Marlatt, & R. J. McMahon (Eds.), *Addictive behaviors across the life span: Prevention, treatment, and policy issues* (pp. 161–183). Newbury Park, CA: Sage.

Brown, S. A., Mott, M. A., & Myers, M. G. (1990). Adolescent drug and alcohol treatment outcomes. In R. R. Watson (Ed.), *Prevention and treatment of drug and alcohol abuse* (pp. 373–403). Clifton, NJ: Humana Press.

Buckley, W. E., Yesalis, C. E. 3rd, Friedl, K. E., Anderson, W. A., Streit, A. L., & Wright, J. E. (1998). Estimated prevalence of anabolic steroid use among male high school seniors. *Journal of the American Medical Association, 260*(23), 3441–3445.

Bukstein, O. G., Glancy, L. J., & Kaminer, Y. (1992). Patterns of affective comorbidity in a clinical population of dually diagnosed adolescent substance abusers. *Journal of the American Academy of Child and Adolescent Psychiatry, 31*, 1041–1045.

CDC. (n.d.). Behavioral Risk Factor Surveillance System Prevalence Data. Atlanta, GA: US Department of Health and Human Services, CDC. Retrieved April 1, 2010, from http://www.cdc.gov/brfss.

CDC. (2007). Web-based Injury Statistics Query and Reporting System (WISQARS). Atlanta, GA: US Department of Health and Human Services, CDC. Retrieved from http://www.cdc.gov/ncipc/wisqars/default.htm

Clark, D., Neighbors, B. (1996). Adolescent substance abuse and internalizing disorders. *Child & Adolescent Psychiatric Clinics of North America, 5*, 45–57.

Cornelius, J. R., Kirisci, L., Reynolds, M., Clark, D. B., Hayes, J., & Tarter, R. (2010). PTSD contributes to teen and young adult cannabis use disorders. *Addictive Behaviors, 35*(2), 91–94.

Crowley, T. J., & Riggs, P. D. (1995). Adolescent substance use disorder with conduct disorder and comorbid conditions. *NIDA Research Monograph, 156*, 49–111.

Dakof, G., Tejeda, M., & Liddle, H. (2001). Predictors of engagement in adolescent drug abuse treatment. *Journal of the American Academy of Child and Adolescent Psychiatry, 40*(3), 274–281.

Deas, D., Riggs, P., Langenbucher, J., Goldman, M., & Brown, S. (2000). Adolescents are not adults: Developmental considerations in alcohol users. *Alcoholism, Clinical and Experimental Research, 24*(2), 232–237.

Deas, D., & Thomas, S. (2001). An overview of controlled studies of adolescent substance abuse treatment. *The American Journal on Addictions, 10*, 178–189.

Dennis, M., Godley, S. H., Diamond, G., Tims, F. M., Babor, T., Donaldson, J., …Funk, R. (2004). The Cannabis Youth Treatment (CYT) study: Main findings from two randomized trials. *Journal of Substance Abuse Treatment, 27*(3), 195–196.

Ehlers, C. L., & Criado, J. R. (2010). Adolescent ethanol exposure: does it produce long-lasting electrophysiological effects? *Alcohol, 44*(1), 27–37.

Fiorentine, R. (1999). After drug treatment: Are 12 step programs effective in maintaining abstinence? *American Journal of Drug and Alcohol Abuse, 25*(1), 93–116.

Fiorentine, R., & Hillhouse, M. P. (2000). Drug treatment and 12 step participation: The additive effects of integrated recovery activities. *Journal of Substance Abuse Treatment. 18*(1), 65–74.

Fleish, B. (1991). Approaches in the treatment of adolescents with emotional and substance abuse problems (DHHS Publication ADM 91–1744). Washington, DC: U.S. Government Printing Office.

Friedman, A. S., & Utada, A. A. (1989). A method of diagnosing and planning the treatment of adolescent drug abusers (the Adolescent Drug Abuse Diagnosis Instrument). *Journal of Drug Education, 19*, 285–282.

Galvez-Buccollini, J. A., DeLea, S., Herrera, P. M., Gilman, R. H., & Paz-Soldan, V. (2009). Sexual behavior and drug consumption among young adults in a shantytown in Lima, Peru. *BMC Public Health, 9*, 23.

Geller, B., Cooper, T. B., Sun, K., Zimerman, B., Frazier, J., Williams, M., & Heath, J. (1998). Double blind placebo controlled study of lithium, for adolescent bipolar disorders with secondary substance dependency. *Journal of the American Academy of Child and Adolescent Psychiatry, 37*(2), 171–178.

Giancola, P. R., Martion, C. S., Tarter, R. E., Pelham, W. E., & Moss, H. B. (1996). Executive functioning and aggressive behavior in preadolescent boys at risk for substance abuse/dependence. *Journal of Studies on Alcohol, 57*, 352–359.

Gibbons, R. D., Hur, K., Bhaumik, D. K., & Mann, J. J. (2006). The relationship between antidepressant prescription rates and rate of early adolescent suicide. *American Journal of Psychiatry, 163*, 1898–1904.

Greenbaum, P. E., Prange, M. E., Friedman, R. M., & Silver, S. E. (1991). Substance abuse prevalence and comorbidity with other psychiatric disorders among adolescents with severe emotional disturbances. *Journal of the American Academy of Child and Adolescent Psychiatry, 30*, 575–583.

Grucza, R. A., Norberg, K. E., & Bierut, L. J. (2009). Binge drinking among youths and young adults in the United States: 1979–2006. *Journal of the American Academy of Child and Adolescent Psychiatry, 48*(7), 679–680.

Hasin, D. S., Keyes, K. M., Alderson, D., Wang, S., Aharonovich, E., & Grant, B. F. (2008). Cannabis withdrawal in the United States: Results from NESARC. *Journal of Clinical Psychiatry, 69*(9), 1354–1363.

Hinckers, A. S., Laucht, M., Schmidt, M.H., Mann, K.F., Schumann, G., Schuckit, M.A., & Heinz, A. (2006). Low level of response to alcohol as associated with serotonin transporter genotype and high alcohol intake in adolescents. *Biological Psychiatry, 1*; *60*(3):282–7.

Hohman, M., & LeCroy, C. W. (1996). Predictors of adolescent AA affiliation. *Adolescence, 31*(122), 339–352.

Hser, Y., Grella, C., Hubbard, R., Hsieh, S., Fletcher, B., Brown, B., & Anglin, D. (2001). An evaluation of drug treatments for adolescents in 4 US cities. *Archives of General Psychiatry, 58*(7), 689–695.

Hsieh, S., Hoffmann, N. G., & Hollister, C. D. (19980. The relationship between pre-, during-, post-treatment factors, and adolescent substance abuse behaviors. *Addictive Behaviors, 23(4),* 477–488. http://www.whitehousedrugpolicy.gov/drugfact/juveniles/juvenile_drugs_ff.html

Jaffe, S. (1990). *Step workbook for adolescent chemical dependency recovery.* Washington, DC: American Academy of Child and Adolescent Psychology.

Joanning, H., Thomas, F., & Quinn, W. (1992). Treating adolescent drug abuse: A comparison of family systems therapy, group therapy and family drug education. *Journal of Marital and Family Therapy, 18,* 345–356.

Johnston, L. D., O'Malley, P. M., Bachman, J. G., & Schulenberg, J. E. (2009). *Monitoring the Future National Results on Adolescent Drug Use: Overview of Key Findings, 2008* (NIH Publication No. 09-7401). Bethesda, MD: National Institute on Drug Abuse.

Johnston, L. D., O'Malley, P. M., Bachman, J. G., & Schulenberg, J. E. (2008). "Various stimulant drugs show continuing gradual declines among teens in 2008, most illicit drugs hold steady." University of Michigan News Service: Ann Arbor, MI. Retrieved October 6, 2010 from http://www.monitoringthefuture.org.

Kaminer, Y., Bukstein, O., & Tarter, R. E. (1991). *The Teen Addiction Severity Index: Rationale and reliability. The International Journal of the Addictions, 26,* 219–226.

Kandel, D. B., Johnson, J. G., Bird, H. R., Weissman, M. M., Goodman, S. H., Lahey, B. B., … Regier, D. A. (1999). Psychiatric comorbidity among adolescents with substance use disorders: Findings from the MECA study. *Journal of the American Academy of Child and Adolescent Psychiatry, 38*(6), 693–699.

Kelly, J. F., & Mayers, M. G. (2007). Adolescents' participation in Alcoholics Anonymous and Narcotics Anonymous: review, implications and future directions. *Journal of Psychoactive Drugs, 39*(3), 259–269.

Kerr, J. M., & Congeni, J. A. (2007). Anabolic-androgenic steroids: Use and abuse in pediatric patients. *Pediatric Clinics of North America, 54*(4), 771–785.

Kershaw, S., Cathcart, R. (2009). Marijuana is gateway drug for two debates. July 17). *New York Times,* p. 1.

Kessler, R. C., McGonagle, K. A., Zhao, S., Nelson, C. B., Hughes, M., Eshleman, S., … Wittchen, H. U. (1994). Lifetime and 12 month prevalence of DSM III-R psychiatric disorders in the United States. *Archives of General Psychiatry, 51,* 8–19.

Kirisci, L., Tarter, R., & Reynolds, M. (2009). The Violence Proneness Scale of the DUSI-R predicts adverse outcomes associated with substance abuse. *American Journal on Addictions, 18*(2), 173–177.

Kuperman, S., Schlosser, S. S., Lidral, J., & Reich, W. (1999). Relationship of child psychopathology to parental alcoholism and antisocial personality disorder. *Journal of the American Academy of Child and Adolescent Psychiatry, 38*(6), 686–692.

Kuzelova, M., Hararova, A., Ondriasova, E., Wawruch, M., Riedel, R., Benedekova, M., … Plakova, S. (2009). Alcohol intoxication requiring hospital admission in children and adolescents: retrospective analysis at the University Children's Hospital in the Slovak Republic. *Clinical Toxicology, 47*(6), 556–561.

Lewinsohn, P. M., Rohde, P., & Seely, J. R. (1996). Adolescent psychopathology: III. The clinical consequences of comorbidity. *Journal of the American Academy of Child and Adolescent Psychiatry, 34,* 510–519.

Lewis, R., Piercy, F., Sprenkle, D., & Trepper, T. (1990). Family based interventions for helping drug abusing adolescents. *Journal of Adolescent Research, 5,* 82–95.

Liao, Y., Tang, J., Ma, M., Wu, Z., Yang, M., Wang, X., … Hao, W. (2010). Frontal white matter abnormalities following chronic ketamine use: a diffusion tensor imaging study. *Brain, 133*(Pt 7), 2115–2122.

Libby, A. M., Brent, D. A., Morrato, E. H., Orton, H. D., Allen, R., & Valuck, R. J. (2007). Decline in treatment of pediatric depression after FDA advisory on risk of suicidality with SSRIs. *American Journal of Psychiatry, 164,* 884–891.

Libby, A. M., Orton, H. D., & Valuck, R. J. (2009). Persisting decline in depression treatment after FDA warnings. *Archives of General Psychiatry, 66,* 633–639.

Maldonado-Devincci, A. M., Badanich, K. A., & Kirstein, C. L. (2010). Alcohol during adolescence selectively alters immediate and long-term behavior and neurochemistry. *Alcohol, 44*(1), 57–66.

Marlatt, G. A., & Gordon, J. R. (1985). *Relapse prevention.* New York, NY: Guilford.

Martin, C. S., Kaczynski, N. A., Maisto, S. A., Bukstein, O. G., & Moss, H. B. (1995). Patterns of alcohol abuse and dependence symptoms in adolescent drinkers. *Journal of Studies on Alcohol, 56,* 672–680.

Mayzer, R., Fitzgerald, H. E., & Zucker, R. A. (2009). Anticipating problem drinking risk from preschoolers' antisocial behavior: evidence for a common delinquency-related diathesis model. *Journal of the American Academy of Child and Adolescent Psychiatry. 48*(8), 820–827.

Merikangas, K. R., Roiusanville, B. J., & Prusoff, B. A. S. (1992). Familial factors in vulnerability in substance abuse. In M. D. Glantz, R. W. Pickens (Eds.). *Vulnerability to drug abuse* (pp. 75–97). Washington, DC: American Psychological Association.

Milberger, S., Biederman, J., Faraone, S. V., Chen, L., & Jones, J. (1997). ADHD is associated with early initiation of cigarette smoking in children and adolescents. *Journal of the American Academy of Child and Adolescent Psychiatry, 36*(1), 37–44.

Miller, G. (1990). *The Substance Abuse Subtle Screening Inventory—adolescent version.* Bloomington, IN: SASSI Institute.

Miller, W. R., & Rollnick, S. (1983). *Motivational interviewing: Preparing people to change addictive behavior.* New York, NY: The Guilford Press.

Millin, R. P. (1996). Comorbidity of substance abuse and psychotic disorders: Focus on adolescents and young adults. *Child and Adolescent Psychiatric Clinics of North America, 5,* 111–122.

Naimi, T. S., Brewer, R. D., Mokdad, A., Clark, D., Serdula, M. K., & Marks, J. S. (2003). Binge drinking among US adults. *Journal of the American Medical Association, 289*(1), 70–75.

National Institute on Alcohol Abuse and Alcoholism, College Students and Drinking, Alcohol Alert No. 29, Bethesda, MD: U.S. Department of Health and Human Services, 1998.

National Survey on Drug Use and Health. (2006). *Substance use treatment need among adolescents 2003–4. The NSDUH report.* Retrieved from http://www.oas.samhsa.gov/nhsda.htm

Niederhofer, H., & Staffen, W. (2003). Comparison of disulfiram and placebo in treatment of alcohol dependence of adolescents. *Drug and Alcohol Review, 22*(3), 295–297.

Noll, R. B., Zucker, R. A., Fitzgerald, H. E., & Curtis, W. J. (1992). Cognitive and motoric functioning of sons of alcoholic fathers and controls: The early childhood years. *Developmental Psychology, 28,* 665–675.

Offer, D., & Schonert-Reichl, K. A. (1992). Debunking the myths of adolescence: Findings from recent research. *Journal of the American Academy of Child and Adolescent Psychiatry, 31*(6), 1003–1014.

Office of Juvenile Justice and Delinquency Prevention. (2005). Drinking in America: Myths, Realities, and Prevention Policy. Washington, DC: U.S. Department of Justice, Office of Justice Programs, Office of Juvenile Justice and Delinquency Prevention. Retrieved August 31, 2010 from http://www.udetc.org/documents/Drinking_in_America.pdf.

Perlman, G., Johnson, W., & Iacono, W. G. (2009). The heritability of P300 amplitude in 18-year-olds is robust to adolescent alcohol use. *Psychophysiology, 46*(5), 962–969.

Perrin, J. M., Friedman, R. A., Knilans, T. K., Black Box Working Group, & Section on Cardiology and Cardiac Surgery. (2008). Cardiovascular monitoring and stimulant drugs for attention-deficit/hyperactivity disorder. *Pediatrics, 122*(2), 451–3.

Project GHB. Retrieved August 31, 2010 from http://www.projectghb.org/

Rahdert, E. (1991). *The adolescent assessment and referral manual* (DHHS Publication ADM-91-1735). Rockville, MD: National Institute on Drug Abuse.

Reich, W., Earls, F., Frankel, O., & Shayka, J. (1993). Psychopathology in children of alcoholics. *Journal of the American Academy of Child and Adolescent Psychiatry, 32,* 995–1002.

Riggs, P. D., Leon, S., Mikulich, S., & Pottle, L. (1998). An open trial of bupropion for ADHD in adolescents with substance use disorders and conduct disorder. *Journal of the American Academy of Child and Adolescent Psychiatry, 37*(12), 1271–1278.

Rockville, M. D., Tarter, R. E., Kirisci, L., Hegedus, A., Mezich, A., & Yanyukov, M. (1994). Heterogeneity of adolescent alcoholism. In T. F. Babor, V. Hesselbrock, R. E. Meyer, & W. Shoemaker (Eds.), *Types of alcoholics: Evidence from clinical, experimental and genetic research* (pp. 172–180). New York, NY: Annals of the New York Academy of Medicine.

Schepis, T. S, & Krishnan-Sarin, S. (2009). Sources of prescriptions for misuse by adolescents: Differences in sex, ethnicity, and severity of misuse in a population-based study. *Journal of the American Academy of Child and Adolescent Psychiatry, 48*(8), 828–836.

Schepis, T. S., & Krishnan-Sarin, S. (2008). Characterizing adolescent prescription misusers: A population-based study. *Journal of the American Academy of Child and Adolescent Psychiatry, 2008; 47*(7), 745–754.

Schuckit, M. A., Smith, T. L., Trim, R. S., Heron, J., Horwood, J., Davis, J., …ALSPAC Study Team (2008). The self-rating of the effects of alcohol questionnaire as a predictor of alcohol-related outcomes in 12-year-old subjects. *Alcohol, 43*(6), 641–646.

Shaffer, D., Fisher, P., Dulcan, M. K., Davies, M., Piacentini, J., Schwab-Stone, M. E., … Regier, D, A. (1996). The NIMH diagnostic interview schedule for children, version 2.3 (DISC-2.3): Description, acceptability, prevalence rates, and performance in the MECA study. *Journal of the American Academy of Child and Adolescent Psychiatry, 35*, 865–827.

Shedler. J., & Block, J. (1990). Adolescent drug use and psychological health: A longitudinal inquiry. *American Psychologist, 45*, 612–630.

Simon, G., Savarino, J., Operskalski, B., & Wang, P. (2006). Suicide risk during antidepressant treatment. *American Journal of Psychiatry, 163*, 41–47.

Stowell, R. J., & Estroff, T. W. (1992), Psychiatric disorders in substance abusing adolescent inpatients: A pilot study. *Journal of the American Academy of Child and Adolescent Psychiatry, 16*, 103–108.

Substance Abuse and Mental Health Services Administration. (2007). Results from the 2006 National Survey on Drug Use and Health: National Findings (Office of Applied Studies, NSDUH Series H-32, DHHS Publication No. SMA 07-4293).

Town, M., Naimi, T. S., Mokdad, A. H., Brewer, R. D. (2006). Health care access among US adults who drink excessively: Missed opportunities for prevention. *Preventing Chronic Disease, 3*(2), A5.

Vik, P. W., Grizzle, K. L., & Brown, S. A. (1992). Social resource characteristics and adolescent substance abuse relapse. *Journal of Adolescent Chemical Dependency, 2*, 59–74.

Webb, J., Baer, P., & Mckelvey, R. (1995). Development of risk profile for intentions to use alcohol among fifth and sixth graders. *Journal of the American Academy of Child and Adolescent Psychiatry, 34*(6), 772–778.

Weed, N. C., Butcher, J. N., & Williams, C. L. (1994). Development of MMPI-A alcohol/drug problems scales. *Journal of Studies on Alcohol, 55*, 296–302.

Weinberg, N. Z., Rahdert, E., Colliver, J., Glantza, M. (1998). Adolescent substance abuse: A review of the past ten years. *Journal of the American Academy of Child and Adolescent Psychiatry, 37*(3), 252–261.

Wells, E. A., Peterson, P. L., Gainey, R. R., Hawkins, J. D., & Catalano, R. F. (1994). Outpatient treatment for cocaine abuse: A controlled comparison of relapse prevention and twelve step approaches. *American Journal of Drug and Alcohol Abuse, 20*, 1–17.

Wilens, T. E. (2004). Attention-deficit/hyperactivity disorder and the substance use disorders: the nature of the relationship, subtypes at risk, and treatment issues. *Psychiatric Clinics of North America, 27*(2), 283–301.

Wilens T. E., Biederman J., Kwon A., Ditterline J., Forkner P., Moore H., Swezey A., ... Faraone SV. (1999). Risk for substance use disorders in youths with child and adolescent onset bipolar disorder. *Journal of the American Academy of Child and Adolescent Psychiatry, 38*(6), 680–685.

Winters, K. C. (1991). *The personal experience screening questionnaire and manual.* Los Angeles, CA: Western Psychological Services.

Winters, K. C., & Henly, G. A. (1989). *The personal experience inventory test and user's manual.* Los Angeles, CA: Western Psychological Services.

Winters, K. C., & Kaminer, Y. (2008). Screening and assessing adolescent substance use disorders in clinical populations. *Journal of the American Academy of Child and Adolescent Psychiatry, 47*(7), 740–744.

Wu, L. T., Ringwalt, C. L., Mannelli, P., & Patkar, A. A. (2008). Prescription pain reliever abuse and dependence among adolescents: a nationally representative study. *Journal of the American Academy of Child and Adolescent Psychiatry, 47*(6), 1020–1029.

Yusko, D. A., Buckman, J. F., White, H. R., & Pandina, R. J. (2008). Alcohol, tobacco, illicit drugs, and performance enhancers: a comparison of use by college student athletes and nonathletes. *The Journal of American College Health, 57*, 281–290.

Glossary

A

Abuse: Defined as addiction, although seen to have lesser criteria to meet the definition.

Addiction: Also known as dependence, addiction is a brain disease resulting from a chronic pattern of drug use characterized by compulsive engagement in drug seeking behaviors, with loss of sense of control, despite harmful consequences.

Alcohol poisoning: Results from consuming large amounts of alcohol in a short period of time. Binge drinking is the most common cause and results in ineffective breathing and impaired blood circulation. This is a medical emergency where 911 calls have to be made.

Alcoholism: Alcohol addiction or dependence, where there is uncontrolled alcohol use with adverse consequences.

B

Binge drinking: For adult males, it is the consumption of five or more drinks in 2 hours and for adult females, four or more drinks in 2 hours. For adolescents, equivalent amounts of alcohol consumed mean more toxic effects.

Black tar: A form of heroin that is primarily available in the western and southwestern United States, with its color varying from dark brown to black.

C

Club drugs: A diverse group of psychoactive compounds that tend to be abused by teens and young adults at a nightclub, bar, rave, or trance scene.

Cognitive Behavior Therapy: Therapy that uses cognitive and behavioral interventions to improve skills and change maladaptive behaviors, which hinder cessation of drug use.

Controlled substance: Substance defined by the Drug Enforcement Agency with varying levels of addictive potential (based on schedules) and medicinal value.

Crack: A cocaine base that comes in a rock crystal that is heated to produce vapors, which are smoked.

The term *crack* refers to the crackling sound produced by the rock as it is heated.

D

Date rape drugs: Drugs used to sedate unsuspecting victims for purposes of sexual advances.

Day program: An intensive outpatient treatment program that relies heavily on milieu as its defining treatment, combined with behavior interventions, and group, individual, and family therapies.

Dependence: A term that applies to addiction, involving drugs with either or both psychological dependence (perception of not being able to live or function without drugs) and physical dependence (tolerance and withdrawal).

Detoxification: Treatment of drug withdrawal symptoms, of which the level of medical supervision varies with the presence of life-threatening conditions or coexisting medical conditions.

Dissociative anesthetic: Drugs primarily used in surgical operations whose effects can include hallucinations.

Diversion: Occurs when prescribed medications with addictive potential are made available to individuals for the sole purpose of getting high.

Downers: Drugs whose primary effect is to induce motor slowing and sedation.

E

Early First Drinking (EFD): EFD occurs when a person consumes his or her first drink between the ages of 12 and 14 years old.

G

Gateway drug: Drug such as cigarettes, alcohol, or cannabis that is used first, before one moves on to more serious drugs like cocaine, heroin, PCP, methamphetamine, etc.

H

Hallucinogen: Drugs causing perceptual experiences that do not exist in actuality, including visual (seeing things) and auditory (hearing things) perceptions.

Harm-reduction approach: Treatment approach that consists of strategies in minimizing the impact of alcohol use and other high-risk behaviors. It operates on the theory that abstinence and minimal harm are goals, but proponents also recognize that any behavior changes that reduce harm are, by themselves, positive outcomes.

High: Street term for being under the influence of drugs.

I

Intoxicated: More sophisticated term for being under the influence of drugs.

L

Level of response: A measure of one's sensitivity to alcohol. Someone with a low level of response would tend to consume more. It is unique to alcohol.

Limit of detection: The lowest level of drug at which an instrument is able to determine its presence.

Limit of quantitation: The lowest level of drug at which its presence cannot be reliably determined.

M

Motivational Enhancement Therapy: A type of evidence-based, non-coercive, and self-centered psychotherapy aimed at increasing the likelihood to change behaviors. As it applies to addiction, Motivational Enhancement Therapy increases the imbalance toward accepting the need to change from drug-seeking to non-using behaviors.

Multisystemic family therapy: Treatment that takes into account broader social relationships including teachers, neighbors, and other social units interacting with the drug-dependent adolescent. The goal is to keep the adolescent in the community in which he lives and keep him in school. This is a very intensive treatment that has been supported to meet the needs of youngsters with multiple issues and legal problems.

O

Off labeling: Use of medications under one of the following conditions: 1) prescription of an FDA-approved medication outside of its recommended dosage (a physician prescribes higher doses than what is recommended for an approved antidepressant), 2) prescription to an individual in a group for whom the drug was not studied (an approved antidepressant for adults being prescribed to adolescents), or 3) prescription of an approved medication for something other than what is was originally intended for (use of antidepressants for anger control instead of depression). This is an acceptable medical practice that requires full disclosure from physicians to parents to ensure that informed consent is obtained.

Overdose: Taking more than what is prescribed or suggested for a medication. It can be intentional or accidental.

P

Physician hopping: A form of drug seeking behavior in which an individual sees multiple doctors to obtain the desired drug of abuse.

Physiologic dependence: Changes in chemical messengers as evidenced by tolerance and withdrawal. Results from longstanding drug use.

Popping: Introducing heroin into the top layers of the skin.

Psychological dependence: Loss of control (obsessive preoccupation) and the need to use a drug without the necessary physiologic change. It is manifested as craving or loss of sense of control over use.

Pyramiding: Increasing doses of steroids through a cycle allowing for doses to be increased 10–40 times the usual dose.

R

Relapse Prevention: A cognitive behavioral treatment approach aimed at developing self-control; identifying triggers in the environment leading to use and relapse; and developing coping skills in dealing with stressors, triggers, and lapses into substance use.

S

Self-medication: The use of drugs, especially the initial use of drugs, to help one cope with problems or in an attempt to treat anxiety, depression, or disordered thoughts.

Sensitivity: The proportion with which the presence of a drug is correctly identified in drug testing,

Short-acting: A brief duration of medication/drug effects, usually inversely related to how long it takes for the body to get rid of it.

Specialty treatment: Treatment received at any of the following types of facilities: hospitals (inpatient only), drug/alcohol rehabilitation facilities (inpatient or outpatient), or mental health centers.

Speedballing: Injecting a combination of cocaine and heroin.

Stacking: The use of multiple steroids at the same time.

Stimulant: Class of medications that is the first line of treatment for ADHD and is not complicated by drug use.

T

Threshold concentration: The level of drug in a sample that meets or exceeds a preestablished cutoff level. A sample with a level above this concentration is said to be positive.

Tolerance: A condition that is marked by the need for an increased amount of the drug abused to achieve the same high or attenuated reinforcing effects at the same amount. Occurs with drug dependence.

Type II alcoholism: Type of alcoholism characterized by onset of alcoholism before age of 25, male gender, and aggression.

U

Use: Attempt at drug use that may not necessarily result in abuse or dependence.

W

Weed: Street name for marijuana.

Withdrawal: Uncomfortable or even painful bodily complaints and signs that exist after drug use is stopped. Occurs with dependence.

Z

Zero tolerance: A requirement that one's blood alcohol level be 0%.

Index

Note: Tables are noted with a *t*.